Entering the Peach Sisterhood

by: Kathy Rodriguez

Table of Contents

Thanks
Prologue
August 24, 2012
The Beginning
How It All Started
8/25—The Next Day
Meeting Dr. Moxley
Nine Days of Waiting
Dating and Other Stuff
09/19/2011—The Big Day
Recovery
What Not to Say
Stage 1a, Grade 2
Hair Loss
Going Back to Work
Faking It
Peaches
Side Effects
November 15, 2012
Why I Relay (blog entry)
Babies
Emergency Visit
Love and Loss
Valentine's Day 2013
Mom
Famous People and Uterine Cancer
Uterine Cancer: Signs and Symptoms
Uterine Cancer: Staging and Basics
What to Do and Where to Go
Epilogue I: Pushing Forward, One Day at a Time
Epilogue II: Getting Better Yet
Credits

Thanks

There are so many, many wonderful people I have to give thanks to. They have been so gracious and so supportive of me, I probably wouldn't have made it through this fight without them. If I have forgotten to mention anyone, please, please forgive me—my memory's not exactly what it used to be!

Many, many thanks to my three fabulous sisters—Paula, Tabita, and Rachel—and awesome brother Ismael, for always being there for me, no matter what, and for constantly encouraging me not to give up. Thank you, too, for reminding me that our dear sweet mother will always be there for me in spirit, and probably kicking my butt if I ever entertained the thought of giving up! And I also must thank my aunt, my cousins, and my nieces and nephews, for doing so many of the little things that made my day. There are too many things to name, but you know what you did. I love you guys…always!!

Ashley: we first met at work way back in May 2009, I had absolutely no way of knowing that you would quickly become one of my best friends. You have been so wonderful! You mean so much to me, you couldn't even possibly begin to know. We have been through so much together, both good and bad, and I hope that you will always be a part of my life. I love you like I love my sisters. Thank you SO MUCH for saving my life that night. I hope we both find the happiness that we seek. (By the way, it's "midget", you silly half-blonde twit.)

Rebecca, you inspired me so much when you got your wonderful first novel published. It has made me realize that anyone can accomplish their dreams, and that hard work truly does pay off!! And thank you for critiquing my early work.

Richard, the love that flows between you and Tipton has truly given me hope. You two have shown me that love is love, period. Thank you for opening up your lives—and that beautiful *Chateau de Claire*—to me. You have truly given me strength to face anything. (P.S.: Thank you for Sundays!)

The *Sunday Patio Party* crowd—Anthony (we short Spaniards gotta stick together!), Harlie (thanks for the trips to the store, even though you were recovering yourself from surgery), Boston (Leos unite!), Dinah (thank you for taking me to OKC!), Slade, Bethany, Reymi, BJ, Eric, and all the other crazies—you guys are insane! Oh my goodness, the things you wild people do just amaze me! But I can't imagine spending my Sunday nights with a better group of people. I love you all, you have no idea just how much.

My former Maples co-workers…what can I say? I couldn't have picked a better group of people to work with. The 3-11 shift was a little bit more interesting with you fine people. Thanks for letting me rant and rave during my initial diagnosis, and for covering for me while I was away. Carrie, Terri, Brandy, Michelle, Abrisha (oh, the questions you came up with!), Dina, Thomas (you still owe me those 6 cookies and 2 Sprites!), Mary, Connie, Chuck, Laci, Tina, and Tiffany: thanks for being there for me when I needed it and accepting me the way I was. I may no longer work with you guys, but I'll never forget what you did for me.

To Dr. Winfrey and the Women's Clinic of Texoma—you are life savers! I can't say enough about you, but please accept my sincere gratitude. Thank you for running all those tests that you felt were necessary and "not being satisfied" until you knew what was happening with my body. If it wasn't for your tenacity, I don't know where I'd be.

To Dr. Katherine Moxley and the gynecologic oncology staff at the Stephenson Cancer Center at the University of Oklahoma—I don't even know where to begin. On September 10, 2012, I walked into your office, sleepy (8 a.m. appointments do that!) and very, very scared, not knowing what to expect. You took me by the hand and were very, very straightforward but compassionate in explaining everything to me. You were very patient with me in answering my questions—and I had plenty of them! You explained how things were going to go, in a manner that was very easy for me to understand. You left no stone unturned! You have taken such good care of me. I wish all doctors and specialists were like you. From the bottom of my heart—and I truly mean this!—thank you. I'll never forget you for the rest of my life.

To the 7th floor nurses and aides at OU Medical Center Presbyterian Tower—thank you so, so much for taking such good, good care of me after my hysterectomy. I felt so afraid, and so alone that night, that no one understood me, not to mention I was in so much pain! You were there for me when I needed something, whether it was food, water, bathroom assistance, pain meds (sorry for calling you so many times in regards to meds…I know it was A LOT!), plugging up my cell phone, or just a hand to hold while I cried, you were always there for me. You showed me so much kindness and generosity and patience and compassion. I know it was your job, but you handled it with such grace. I wish I could remember all of your names, so I can thank each of you individually. But alas, thank you—always. I hope that I never have to go back, but if I do, I'll know that I'll be in good hands.

Susan—thank you doesn't even begin to describe how I feel. I sincerely appreciate the food, the books, the desserts, and the encouraging words you gave me. You knew exactly how I felt early on, going through this journey, because you have been there. I know I am not in this fight alone. We need more friends like you in this world. I love you to no end.

To those I didn't mention by name—don't think your actions aren't appreciated. Whether it was a dinner, taking out my trash, or anything else, rest assured I'm extremely grateful, and I always will be. I love you forever.

To God Almighty—with You, all things are possible. Your healing hands have provided me with the strength I have needed to fight this deadly disease. Thank You so much.

Finally, to my fellow "peach sisters" who have lost the fight, and those who are still fighting: only you can truly understand the significance of this terrible disease. I will always continue to fight with you and for you. Much love and God bless…always. *Until there is a cure.*

...klr

Prologue

When I first got diagnosed with uterine cancer, I had so many mixed-up thoughts and emotions, I had no idea where to begin. What the hell was I going to do? How in the world was I going to tell people? I was so scared. I didn't know how I was going to handle this. I felt like my life was over, that I wasn't going to cope with this very well.

Then someone suggested that I keep a journal about my cancer fight. *Hmm*, I thought to myself. *That's not a bad idea.* I could totally do something like that. I had so many thoughts rumbling around in my head, I felt it would be beneficial to put them to paper. Then later on, I could look back on my thoughts and see how they have changed.

As I started to write in the journal, I noticed that a lot of these thoughts could be made public, as in starting a blog. A lot of my friends and family had been asking how I was doing and how I was feeling. To keep everyone up to date on my treatment and my fight, I began a blog called "Kathy's Cancer Journey" in September 2012.

Not long after I started my blog, my friend Rebecca became a published author. I was so proud of her that she got her book "out there"! But it did gently remind me of a long-ago dream of mine that I wanted to be a writer. I was a journalism major in college. I had worked for the student newspaper and wrote a few articles, which I have framed and put on my wall. But it's not the same as writing a book and getting published in that manner. So when Rebecca's book got published, it woke up a small part of me that I had thought wasn't there anymore. But what could I write about in this book? Then a post in my online support group on Facebook gave me that final push. I could write about my fight against this terrible disease. I felt that I could provide some sort of inspiration to at least one woman who is just now going through what I did and has the same fears and anxieties. And if I have helped one person by telling my story, then I will most definitely have succeeded.

What you are about to read is my journey—from initial diagnosis to the road of recovery, not to mention other facets of my life. I still have a long way to go from here, but thanks to the love and support of so many wonderful, kick-ass people, I know I am not in this fight alone. And I want you—yes, you!—to know that you aren't alone in this fight, either.

...klr

August 24, 2012

It's Friday today. It's 1:57 p.m., and I'm getting ready for work. I was coming back from two days off, but I was not wanting to go back. I wanted to stay home and sleep. I suppose there's something about having more than one consecutive day off that makes you feel like staying in bed. But anyway…I digress.

That day was just like any other day. It was warm outside, but it was sunny, like Texas usually is this time of year. I was feeling good. I even remember what I was wearing: lavender T-shirt with the State of Texas seal, blue jean shorts, white socks, and Nike sneakers. Funny how I am able to remember stuff like that. I can recall exactly what I was doing when the phone rang. I had just finished putting on my make-up and was about to put on my eye shadow (it was purple—to match the shirt) when my ringtone began blaring. I had dropped my tube of eye shadow on the phone, and somehow, that made the phone pick up. (Damn smart phones. They tend to work when you don't want them to.)

It was Dr. Winfrey's office on the other end of the line. The lady's name was Rebecca or Rachel or something like that. She told me that the results from my two tests had come back. I had forgotten about them. Oh. Oops. That tends to happen to me sometimes—being forgetful. Anyway, she told me that my Pap smear came back normal, so that was a relief. But the next few words are words that I will never forget for the rest of my life: "We also got the results of your biopsy back, and it shows that you do have uterine cancer."

I began crying and almost dropped the phone. Holy hell! I just could not believe it. I didn't WANT to believe it. Who wants to hear a cancer diagnosis at the age of 32? I sure as hell didn't. I had celebrated (if you can call it that) my 32nd birthday just two weeks before. I was most *definitely* not ready for this. No way.

Absolutely not.

I was 32 years old, in the prime of my life: I had a (reasonably) good job I loved with wonderful co-workers, a great family, awesome friends, and a man that I had more than a passing interest in. (I had wanted to see where that might lead.) There was absolutely no room for cancer. *None.* But there it was. Those were the thoughts that were running through my mind as I was on the phone. Six minutes, 30 seconds that changed my life. Six lousy, frickin' minutes. Dammit!

As I stayed on the phone, the words "uterine cancer" kept repeating themselves over and over in my head. It didn't seem like it was real. It was like someone's idea of a cruel joke. Well, I didn't think it was funny at all. I tried concentrating on the words the nurse was telling me. "It's a very curable type of cancer," she said to me. "We're certain that we found it early and in time to do something to keep it from spreading." Okay, I suppose that was my silver lining in all of this. But still, hearing those words can do something to a person. You are never, ever the same after that. So many thoughts and emotions are going through your mind: fear, anger, hostility, resentment, just to name a few. You wonder why this has happened to you, what you did to deserve this. You begin to think about your life up to that point. And that's what I started to do with mine. I started to look back at what I had done in the previous 32 years. And when I started thinking about my life, I had no idea it would lead to this life-altering incident.

...klr

The Beginning

    My life started out pretty normal. I was born in a small north Texas town (15 minutes from the Texas-Oklahoma border) on a hot August afternoon in 1980. My mother would later tell me that 1980 was considered to be the hottest summer on record. (I have to disagree with that—July and August 2011 are right up there as far as heat goes!) I was the youngest child my mother had. I had three living sisters (another one, Elisabeth, died in 1962 as an infant) and a brother, and they were all older than me, by a considerable margin. (My youngest sister, Rachel, is 12 years older than me, and my sister Paula already had two kids when I was born.) My mother was 39 years old when she had me—and was in her early to mid-20's when she had my siblings. So, um, yeah…I was most definitely unintended, to say the least. My father (or, shall I say, "sperm donor") was 20 years older than my mother—yeah, I know…ICK!! You would think that since he was so much older than her, he would somehow feel sort of responsibility towards me. But no, it didn't happen that way. He left my mother the moment he found out she was pregnant, as so many men do in these situations, and never came back. So much for being a father. I have never met him, and I never want to, either. Why should I? He's never wanted anything to do with me, and he's never made any amount of effort to see me. The way I figure it, if he truly wanted to be a part of my life, he would have done it already. So I don't miss him at all. (How can you miss someone you've never met?) My mom did an awesome job by herself. She was both mother and father to me, and I turned out just fine, thank you very much.

    For the longest time, it was just the two of us, me and my mom. There were a lot of times that we struggled. She survived an abusive and alcoholic husband, a health scare when I was 12, and raised me almost completely on her own. She left her last husband (I absolutely refuse to call him my stepfather—to me, he never earned that right) after she found out he molested me on a weekly basis for almost two years. Why did my mom stay with him for so long? Well, she didn't know about the sexual abuse. I was too afraid to tell her. That old adage, about how victims believe that the abuse is their fault and that they somehow caused this to happen to them, it's true. But I finally got up the courage to spill my guts. My mother, bless her heart, left her husband, and we started a new life on our own. We moved from Brenham, Texas to where I live now, to be closer to the rest of our family. It was not easy by any stretch of the imagination (we struggled a lot), as I have said, but my mother was an extremely tough woman, and if she wanted to do something, well, dammit, she did it.

She started getting sick towards the end of my senior year of high school in 1999. I was sad, because I thought it meant that I couldn't go to college, like I had wanted. It had been my dream to attend the University of North Texas and major in sports journalism, and I had just been accepted there—free ride and everything. I thought I had to give up my dream and stay home to take care of her. But my sweet mother insisted that I go to college; that's how tough she was…she didn't want to be a burden to me. "Besides," she had told me, "I have the rest of the family to help me." So off to UNT I go, and I was there for two wonderful years, but I still worried about her, so I transferred to Midwestern State University, which was only 45 minutes away (compared to the three hours of UNT), so that I could be closer to her, if she ever needed anything. I was at MSU for a semester before my mom got really sick, so I left college completely so that I could take care of her. I still intend to get my bachelor's degree someday, but I want to take care of some things first (like beating cancer!) before I do. Anyway, I took care of my mom for the next 5 ½ years until September 2007.

She had just finished yet another hospital stint (she had a lot of those—she didn't take care of herself for years), and the doctor wanted her to get some extended rehab therapy at the nursing home. I had just started my job at the state hospital the month before. Unfortunately, I had to admit that I could no longer work and take care of my mom. I didn't know what to do. I couldn't (nor did I want to, to be honest) quit the job, but on the other hand, I wanted and needed to take care of my mom, too. She meant the world to me. But my mother, bless her, took matters into her own hands. She decided to turn the temporary stay in the nursing home into a permanent one. "You need to live your own life now," she said when I asked her why she was doing this. "I want you to enjoy your job. You've worked hard for it. And I want you to find someone one day and settle down. You can't do that if you're taking care of me." And so she lived the next 18 months as a very contented woman.

My mother began to die a very slow and painful death. It was the one thing she did not want to do. She didn't want any tubes inserted to keep her living, and in the end, she didn't have them. But for almost 8 months, she did have them, to drain away all the infections she had developed in those final months. Finally, all the tubes she was attached to were removed, as was her wish. She said if she was going to die, it was going to be "without those damn wires" (her words). She struggled to survive for so long, it was painful and hard to watch. It was heartbreaking, too, because I was helpless. I couldn't help her, like I had done so many times in the past. She was hurting, and hurting so much. She just wanted to stop hurting. "I can't fight no more," she would tell me on more than one occasion. "I want to go home. See my baby Lisa and my momma." This wonderful woman fought as long as she could, but in the end, even she couldn't fight anymore. She lost her long battle on December 31, 2009, at the age of 68. She always said she was going to go on her own terms, and sure enough, she did. And when she died, she left behind a strong legacy. Those that were blessed to come across her in their lives never forgot her, she had that much of an impact. She instilled in me a willingness, stubbornness, and determination to fight for everything I believed in. It's that fighting spirit that has gotten me through this particular journey. It's because of her that I absolutely refuse to give up. I'm gonna get through this. My mother would not want it any other way.

...klr

How It All Started

My memory's not what it used to be (I suppose that's a result of being hit in the head at work), so there aren't too many things that I can remember too well. But I can definitely remember—clear as day!—how my cancer fight got started and the medical emergency that ultimately led to my diagnosis.

I had bad monthly cycles for 8-plus years, after the car accident I had in July 2004, where I overturned 3 times at 70mph on I-45 outside Huntsville, Texas…in the rain, no less. Doctors said I was lucky to be alive. "WHY aren't you dead?", one of them kept repeating. Great bedside manner, doc! But I digress…before then, I did not have one single issue with my periods. Each month since I was 11 years old, I had had a monthly cycle—on the 17th of each month, without fail and like clockwork. But after the accident, the cycles went berserk. I didn't have any for the first 5 years, then, on and off, for three years after that, I had sporadic cycles. *Why didn't you go to the doctor sooner?*, you ask. I had one simple reason—I had no health insurance. And without insurance, health care can get mighty expensive. Besides, I had no real desire to go. But anyhow, I started to have somewhat regular cycles for about six months (though I had really heavy ones, but I didn't concern myself with that minor detail). I was excited, for sure. It meant that I might be able to have kids after all. And that was something I was truly looking forward to. Woo hoo and all that.

I can pinpoint the exact day that my recent issues started. I began my period on July 20, 2012. At first I was excited, but then I got mad because that was the exact day that I was starting my vacation with my sister Rachel and my two nephews. Honestly, who really wants to start a vacation during "that" time of the month? I knew I most certainly didn't, that was for damn sure! I remember settling into the hotel in San Antonio that first night, and I spent a little too much time in the restroom. After my sister used the restroom, she asked me, "Umm, Kathy, are you on your period? I saw the toilet paper you used." (Our mother taught us to wrap our used feminine pads with TP before throwing them away in the trash.) "Don't remind me," I said glumly. "Oh, that sucks," she said. "Maybe it will last a few days and then you can enjoy the rest of the vacation." That was my hope, but psshh. It didn't happen that way. I ended up being on my cycle for the entire nine days of the vacation. Hah! Some vacation, Mother Nature! Thanks a lot! I had taken a box and a half of feminine pads with me, and I came back with just three measly pads. Not good, but certainly not the end of the world. I could always buy more. Anyhow, I continued to have my period for several days after coming back home. Hmm, ok, this is not a good thing. "Dammit!" I would tell myself on more than one occasion. But I still didn't want to visit a doctor. Why? Well, in addition to inheriting my mother's fighting spirit, I inherited her stubborn streak, too. If I didn't want to do something, I didn't do it, just like her. It was hard to get me to a doctor of any type. I was kinda hoping the problem would go away on its own. But it didn't. It just kept flowing and flowing. I didn't want these problems. And it only got worse. At times, the flow and cramping would be so bad that I would be in tears and doubled over in pain. I had so much trouble sleeping from all the pain. Even the strongest of medicines didn't help. I prayed for God to take away my pain. I hated feeling this way. But finally one day the flow appeared to stop. It was as if someone had turned off a faucet or something. I was so happy, so excited. But my happiness did not last very long.

I started again the very next day, August 14th. It had started off as a light flow. OK, I told myself, I can deal with this. No big deal. Hakuna matata and all that. I was at work when it began (thankfully I was wearing a pad as a precaution), and I was needing to eat and take my meds, so I went on break at about six p.m. I went to the restroom and noticed that the flow had gotten somewhat heavier, so I changed my pads, cleaned up and finished my break. Ten minutes after returning from my break, I felt something *pop* down there. Oh, no, I thought to myself. Then I began to feel something flow hard, as if someone had poured a drink down a drain or something like that. I had asked my boss Lori for permission to go home and change. "What's wrong?" she asked me. "Um, it's that time of the month, and I need to change *now*," I whispered to her. "The blood has soaked through my shorts. Please let me go. I'll be back as soon as I can. I promise." "Well, okay," she told me. "Just take your time and make sure everything's all right before you come back." I rushed out of the security gate at 7:40 in the evening and went straight home as fast as I could, in spite of the rain that had just started coming down. When I arrived at my apartment, I went straight to the bathroom, which was a good thing, because I narrowly escaped losing consciousness from the excessive amount of blood loss. To this day, it amazes me how I was able to drive 1.5 miles to my apartment with blurry vision and a monster headache, in the rain. (It was a small miracle that I did. I like to think that it was God— and my mom—watching over me and protecting me.)

I sat down on the toilet and the flow that came out of me, like water coming out of a fire hydrant when something hits it. I could not believe it was flowing that hard, but I thought I was urinating. *Nah, that can't be right*, I told myself. *I just used the restroom on break, and I didn't drink anything to be peeing like this. I shouldn't be going again so soon. Something* has *to be wrong*. So I got myself cleaned up and changed, and I was ready to go back to work. I looked in the toilet before flushing it to see what had happened. Oh my god, I could not believe my eyes! I saw nothing but dark red water. I had never been so, so petrified in my entire life. No wonder I was feeling light-headed. My dear sweet friend Ashley (I owe her my life, now that I think about it), who I happened to be texting at the time at the time, made me go to the emergency room, and simply wouldn't take "no" for an answer. I spent two hours in that godforsaken place. My nerves were shot, and on top of that, the power had gone out because of the thunderstorm. (I am severely claustrophobic—the power outage did NOT help.) It just wasn't my day. The doctor—I forget his name—told me he would do a pelvic exam. "It's gonna hurt a little," he tells me right before he inserts the instrument. "HOLY SHIT!" I screamed at him. "A little?! It's like you're ripping out my insides!!" But the exam was over almost as soon as it began, thank the Lord. "Well," he says, "there's no tearing. So you're not bleeding from that." He ordered some blood work, but that didn't reveal anything either. "Do you have a gynecologist?" he asked after the blood work came back. "No," I tell him. "I do have an appointment set up with someone in October, though." "Sweetheart," he tells me, "you can't afford to wait that long. Go in the next couple of days." I called the gynecologist's office the next morning and got my October 30th appointment moved up to the next day, the 16th of August. Wow, that was rather quick.

So I met Dr. Winfrey that next day, the 16th of August, and she couldn't have been more wonderful to me. "I'm gonna do a Pap smear and get some tissue samples from your uterus, see if we can't figure out why you're bleeding so much," she explains. "They're gonna be a little uncomfortable but they're not gonna take that long." She was right…nothing to it. And they were A LOT better to endure than that damn pelvic exam. Eight days later, I was given the horrible news that I had uterine cancer. I had so many emotions: sadness, anger, resentment, emotional…to name a few. But to be honest, I was relieved, too. Why is that? Because I finally knew what the hell was going on, and it wasn't just my imagination. It also meant that I could finally begin my road to recovery.

To be honest, I don't remember most of these days, especially the 14th. Most of what I just mentioned was based on what others have told me that I communicated to them. It's amazing how I still don't have a recollection of what happened. Perhaps it's a mental block. Whatever it was, these events helped change my life—dramatically.

…klr

8/25—The Next Day

It's now been a full 24 hours since my cancer diagnosis, and the news still affects me. At any given moment, I would spontaneously burst into tears. My co-workers had picked up on the fact that something wasn't quite right with me. I didn't know exactly how to break the terrible news to them. It's not exactly something you bring up in a normal conversation. But I finally managed to say those few difficult words: "I have cancer. I just found out yesterday." To say they were shocked and dismayed was an understatement. I do believe they ached for me. A couple of them cursed, some said, "oh, honey, I'm so sorry!", some hugged me, some (I think) might have kicked something, and I think one guy turned white and slammed a door (I think he might have taken it the hardest).

The awesome thing about my fellow co-workers is that they were there for me at a time when I needed them the most. They hugged me, they comforted me, and they made me laugh; but most of all, they let me be "me". They didn't try to change me, which I appreciate. They let me carry on and on. I couldn't have asked for a better group of humans. Yes, we have had our moments, but I truly care about them. I sincerely mean that in every way. Honestly, I don't know what I could have done without them. I was truly blessed, and I couldn't have asked for much more than that.

…klr

Meeting Dr. Moxley

I was not expecting Dr. Winfrey's office to call me again so soon after giving me my cancer diagnosis. But they did. They called me on the 27th, the Monday after telling me I had cancer. It was the same young woman that had called me the first time. During the first phone call, she had told me I had more than one option about where I wanted to go for treatment. "We don't have any specialists here in Wichita Falls that deal with uterine cancer," she'd said. "So we're going to let you choose where you want to go. You can go to Dallas, or you can go to Oklahoma City. Both have excellent doctors, and in either case, you will be in very good hands." Well, I don't really like Dallas roads all that much (I hate them, actually), and I had never been to Oklahoma City, so OKC was my choice.

When Dr. Winfrey's office called me back that following Monday, I figured that I'd be told the OKC specialist was not accepting any new patients. But that wasn't the case. (They're always accepting patients—cancer never stops.) "We've got an appointment set up for you to see Dr. Moxley in Oklahoma City," the nurse said. She told me that my appointment was on September 10th, which was only two weeks from that day. Wow, I couldn't believe I was going to see a cancer specialist so soon. Getting an appointment with a doctor like that usually took forever. (I once had to wait three months to see an ear, nose, and throat specialist.) But I guess the severity of my situation warranted speedy arrangements. I requested and received time off from work, and off to Oklahoma City I go.

I took my sister Tabita and my aunt Mickey with me to the appointment. We left for the trip the afternoon before because my appointment was scheduled for 8 a.m. Monday morning, and the drive would take three hours, and there was no way in hell I was getting up early to drive that far. (I had enough issues to deal with!) Getting to Oklahoma City wasn't as hard as I thought it would be, though. The scenery helped me a lot. We got settled into the hotel at about four in the afternoon and rested a while. Before I turned in for the night, I took a shower. I guess the emotions of the previous two weeks finally got to me, because I just started sobbing like crazy, and I couldn't stop. I became angry with God, though I know I shouldn't have done so. "Why me, God?!" I cried out. "Why did you do this to me? Why did you give me cancer? I didn't do anything to anyone to deserve this." But I began to realize that it wasn't God's fault—or anyone else's fault, for that matter. No one *gives* you cancer. It just happens. And no one deserves any type of disease. That's just how life is sometimes.

This was the thought that was running through my mind as I went to bed that night. I couldn't sleep very well, so I was awake at 4:45 a.m. Yup, I was that nervous. I got ready and ate a honey bun for breakfast. I remember checking out of the hotel after everyone had finished getting ready. Oh, goodness, the air was cold! Where did the cold weather come from? It certainly wasn't cold the day before. I was nervous, I was cold, I was hungry, and I was sleepy.

I had never been to Oklahoma City before, so I was a bit apprehensive about driving through the streets, especially since it was morning rush hour. But believe it or not, the roads were easy to navigate, and I got to the cancer center in no time at all.

I drove onto the campus of OU Health Sciences Center bright and early. Hmm, a campus, I thought to myself. This is good…means that these people are always doing some kind of research in the health care field and patients will be the beneficiaries of that extensive studying and research. I pulled into the parking garage of the Stephenson Cancer Center, and I was amazed at the sheer size of the building. Good Lord, this place was huge! It was beautiful, though—the place was easily 6 stories tall. So many windows! The inside of the building was just as nice—so many plush couches and chairs, and so many books and magazines to read! It looked like a rich person's private library more than a doctor's office. It didn't look like anything I had expected. I suppose that was a good thing—when you're at an oncologist's office for the first time, you're going through so many emotions, and the staff wants you to be as comfortable as possible.

It didn't take long from the time I arrived to the time I was taken to an exam room—an advantage to having an 8 a.m. appointment. The nurse's assistant asked me several questions about my overall health and took my vital signs—even my weight! (I hate being weighed!) I was then taken to a meeting where I was given something to drink, and I met a physician's assistant—his name was Kenneth—and another woman, who was probably a resident. Kenneth's questions were more in-depth. I hated answering them in the presence of my sister and my aunt. There are just some things you don't want your family to know and hear about, especially if those issues were gynecologic in nature. Talk about embarrassing. The questions and answers took about 30 minutes.

I was left alone in the room with my sister and my aunt for a few minutes. Like I said, I was nervous—just a little. I was wondering if Dr. Moxley was any good, if she was as good as advertised. I knew absolutely nothing about her—didn't know her personality, her demeanor, what she looked like, what her record of accomplishment was, if she was any good at this sort of thing—not a thing. The fact that I didn't know how far my cancer had advanced did not help matters at all.

The door opened, and three women walked in—the resident from before, plus two others, one a tall beautiful blonde, and the other one a short brunette, but just as pretty. She was ok, but I didn't know about her. She looked kinda young to be working in this field. I figured that the tall blonde was going to be Dr. Moxley and the short brunette was her assistant or something like that. But I was way off-base. "Which one of you is Kathy?" asked the short brunette. I meekly raised my arm and she stuck her hand out. "Hi, I'm Dr. Moxley, and this is Dr. Bishop," she told me, referring to the blonde. "She'll be helping me." Wow…could have fooled me! I totally had that all wrong. Dr. Moxley was a petite woman, who barely measured 5 feet in height. (I highly suspected her shoes might have put her over that mark.) She looked kinda young, too…early to mid-30's. But to be honest, this didn't bother me much. As long as she cured me, I didn't give a damn what she looked like.

Dr. Moxley began to explain what type of uterine cancer I had (endometrial adenocarcinoma), and what she wanted to do. What impressed me about this incredibly awesome woman was that she didn't try to rush me. She took the time to explain how things happened and how things were going to go for me. There were so many things I didn't understand and so many questions I had to ask. (After all, this was my health.) She took the time and answered each question slowly, thoughtfully, and carefully. She was very straightforward but very compassionate at the same time, something that isn't exactly easy to do. After our initial meeting, she did an ultrasound to see where everything was. I was told that it was going to be uncomfortable, but honestly, it wasn't. I got to see everything, which was cool. Dr. Moxley even pointed out where the cancer was located. It looked like it was located on the endometrium, the part of the uterine wall that helps protect a fetus when a woman is pregnant. She explained that this most likely meant the cancer was caught very, very early. She was open to doing chemo and radiation, then surgery because of my age, to preserve fertility. She also explained, "it would be better to do the hysterectomy." How come? Can't you just keep an eye on it? "No," she said. "It's not the type of situation where we just sit back and keep an eye on it. It's manageable, but it's also significant. We have to take it out as soon as possible." She also explained that there were several cysts on my ovaries (but they weren't cancerous, which was good), so those had to be taken out as well. I cried because what all of this meant was that I would never have any kids. I kinda had a feeling this would happen from the moment I received my diagnosis, but it hurt to hear this come from my doctor. But as long as I was healthy, that was all that mattered.

Dr. Moxley and I then made plans to do the total hysterectomy and salpingo-oopherectomy (removal of the ovaries). She wanted to do it on the 12th of September, as soon as possible. Umm, no. That was *way* too soon—only two days away. And it was my aunt's birthday. I didn't want her to have that memory on her birthday. Besides, I needed to get a few things in order. So we instead decided to do the surgery on the following Wednesday; September 19th. That gave me enough time to get things organized at work. Dr. Moxley also explained that she would remove several lymph nodes, so she could determine whether or not chemo and/or radiation were necessary. She also explained how long I was going to be out of work. Four weeks minimum, she said. Psshh. All that time doing absolutely nothing. Boy, was I going to be bored out of my mind!

  I finally got to leave Oklahoma City a little after 3:30 p.m. It was easily the longest day of my life. But I went home a happy woman. I met the most amazing doctor, and she made me feel at ease. I knew that I was going to be ok…I was in good hands. Dr. Moxley may have been short in stature, but that was ok. She was a very smart, caring woman and knew what the hell she was doing. Can't ask for more than that.

…klr

Nine Days of Waiting

     After I got home from Oklahoma City, all I could do was wait til the 19th. I wish I could have made the time go by faster, because I wanted to get this mess over with. I have a serious aversion to hospitals—I spent so much time in them with my mom when she was sick. I didn't like being helpless, either, and being in a hospital meant that I was going to be helpless for a while, and that I was gonna have to be dependent on others. (I was a very independent person.) So many thoughts and emotions were going through my mind. I have the tendency to think the worst, especially when it comes to stuff like this. I kept thinking that something was going to go wrong while I was on the operating table. I also kept thinking I was going to get bad hospital care. Deep down, I knew things were going to go smoothly, but I couldn't help but feel like panicking.

     My emotions weren't any better after my initial visit. If anything, they were probably worse. I still had the tendency to spontaneously burst into tears. It was hard to do nothing but sit back and wait, to sit back and let cancer sit in your system. I wanted to get rid of my cancer. I didn't know how much I had, and I didn't know if it had spread beyond the uterine wall. I was also afraid of the possibility of having to do chemo and/or radiation. Dr. Moxley told me that there was only a 50% chance of needing further treatment post-hysterectomy. I had heard how chemotherapy and radiation had horrible, horrible side effects, and I didn't want to experience any of the nausea or vomiting or anything else like that. Besides, I didn't know if they were going to be effective or not. My friend Susan had breast cancer in 2011, and needed both radiation and the chemo. She lost her hair and energy early, and she was sick a lot. I did not want that to happen to me. I was already gonna be out for a significant amount of time from work—6 to 8 weeks. (So much for only being out for 4 weeks!) I didn't want to be out longer than that. I loved my job, and my co-workers and patients meant the world to me, and being away from them was gonna sting. I also tend to be vain about my hair. If I was going to require the chemotherapy and radiation, I was going to be losing all of it. I liked my hair; I wanted to keep it.

My co-workers, bless them, tried their absolute best to make me feel better about my diagnosis and my course of treatment. One of them, Abrisha, just blew me away with the things she would suggest. "What are they taking out?" she would ask me. Everything, I would answer. "Everything? Even the eggs?" Umm, yeah, even the eggs. The tubes, too. "Damn! That means you'll never have any babies." Yup, that's pretty much it, Abrisha. "Well, that sucks. I'm sorry. Look at it this way, though. You'll get to have all the sex you want, all day long, and you don't ever have to worry about getting pregnant." I was extremely sensitive around this time about having children, and any comment about this subject caused lots and lots of tears. But something about the way she had said it made me laugh—it was too funny.

Like I said, I was also a bit sensitive about potentially losing my hair. Two of my absolutely wonderful co-workers, Thomas and Chuck, made me laugh one night as we were leaving work. I was feeling kinda bummed (again) about the chemo and radiation, and of course the hair loss. These guys are wonderful, and the women they are with are lucky, indeed. But anyway, I had said I didn't see how losing my hair was a good thing. "Just think of all the money you'll be saving by not having to buy shampoo and stuff," Chuck tells me. Yeah, I suppose that's true, I say. "And think of all the cool hairstyles you could have," Thomas says to me. "Be whatever you want. You could be blonde, or you could have hot pink hair, or make it electric blue. Better yet, you could even have a stripper wig." Umm, what? "A stripper's wig, kinda like what a stripper would wear during one of her shows. You could pretend to be a stripper!" Umm, no, I think I'll pass, I tell him. I'll stick to the hot pink tresses, thank you very much.

My two friends Carrie and Terri helped me, too. They gave me more hugs and more words of encouragement than anyone else did. The pep talks they gave me during those nine days are of a private nature, so I won't reveal what was said. But they helped me tremendously, they have no idea.

I had so many friends and family take me out to eat, text or call me, or just generally let me hang out with them. I revealed my innermost thoughts and fears and anxieties, and they just let me carry on. They let me know that everything was going to be okay, and that I was not alone. They were always gonna be there for me. Always.

...klr

Dating and Other Stuff

Your life changes dramatically once you have a hysterectomy, especially if it's a total one, like the one I had. You don't feel like a complete woman anymore, and you have nothing to offer anybody. You can't have kids, so what else are you able to do for a guy?

I have always been an extremely shy person in front of guys, especially those that I like and have feelings for. I suppose that stems from my abusive childhood, and being completely uncomfortable around guys. I couldn't stand the thought of letting a guy near me, my self-esteem was that bad. It did get better for me in college, though. I actually dated a couple of guys, even becoming engaged to one of them. But I wasn't ready for marriage, I don't think. Honestly, who's ready for marriage at 19? It's hard when a relationship ends, and you feel like a failure. So there went my self-esteem again.

For the longest time, I had been wanting to find a guy and settle down with him, maybe have kids somewhere down the line. But it seemed that no one was ever really interested in me. I am not the most beautiful person in the world, and I don't look like one of those stick-thin models you see on television and in movies and magazines. I'll never, ever be a size 2, or anything close to that, no matter how hard I try to lose the weight. But I am a wonderful person to be with, and I am very, very loyal to those I love. What I lack in beauty, I more than make up for in personality. But most (if not all) of the guys that I show a slight interest in never notice me. They usually show an interest in other people. And that's just too bad. These guys are truly missing out, my friends tell me. That may be true, but it doesn't help my self-esteem any when I see the guy I care about develop feelings for someone else, especially if she's prettier than me.

I even tried one of those online dating sites one time to find somebody. I was even successful—I found a guy who actually showed a little interest in me. We were together for a while. But for some reason, it just didn't work out, and I haven't been in a true relationship since then. Lame, I know. There was also someone that I had an intense interest in a few years back. One might even venture to say that I was in love with him. In hindsight, I suppose I was. But some things happened, and I was greatly betrayed. Apparently, he didn't feel the same about me that I did about him. Perhaps he did, I don't know. If he did, he had a lousy way of showing it. But now that I've had time to think about it, maybe he didn't do such a bad job of showing how he truly felt about me. I just refused to see it. I was just not used to having a guy that was actually interested in *me* and wanted to be with me and *only me,* and actually thought I was beautiful. My self-esteem still sucked back then. I couldn't imagine what he wanted with me, so I guess I did my absolute best to push him away. He was a patient guy, but even patient people have their limits. And I apparently reached his.

In hindsight, I am actually glad it didn't work out between the two of us. I realize now that we were totally mismatched. The relationship would have been doomed from the beginning. And it's better to be single than to be in a bad and toxic relationship, I would think. It would not have been good for me—or for him, for that matter. And we both deserve better.

My friend Ashley used to tell me that I'm just too picky and that I'm just afraid of getting hurt again. And she's right—I am. But I have tried to get better about all of it. For the most part, I don't think I'm as picky as I once was. Opening up to someone—that's a little bit harder to do still. I've tried to be more receptive to guys, but it's not coming to me naturally. I still think they're going to hurt me. It all comes down to my self-esteem, or lack thereof. And now that I've had cancer and the hysterectomy, my overall well-being has really taken a hit. I can't offer a guy the chance to one day have children. For most guys, that's a deal-breaker.

Having this hysterectomy has made me confront the possibility that I may end up alone for the rest of my life. And that's not something I am looking forward to at all.

...klr

09/19/2012—The Big Day

It seemed like it would take forever, but the day of my surgery finally arrived. It was funny, though—I had been so ready for this day, but now that it had arrived, I kinda wanted those nine days back. I didn't know what was ahead for me, and that scared me. I didn't have any control over what was happening to me. I was so used to being able to plan things for myself. Getting cancer was not on the agenda at all!

But now that the day was here, I might as well face it. I tried preparing for it the best way I could. Honestly, though, who can effectively prepare for something like this? Truth is, you can't.

I had plenty of wonderful support from people in my life. My family started helping me around the apartment, which I totally appreciated. They helped me clean up, throw away my trash, and bought me food or drinks. My friends and people from work helped me tremendously, too. The last couple of days that I was at work before I went on medical leave, I was given so many well wishes and so many hugs, I had enough to last a very long time!

I had three days off from work before I had my surgery. You would think that I would use that time to take care of any last-minute things. Psshh. As if. I slept on and off a lot and I had a late lunch with my friend Ashley that ended up lasting five hours. (We were there so long we got kicked out when they closed for the night.) But I did pack my suitcase and got all my paperwork together. I just didn't organize my apartment the way I wanted.

I left for Oklahoma City the day before my surgery with my sister Tabita. We got to OKC fairly early, so we went sightseeing downtown. We got to tour the Oklahoma State Capitol, which was awesome—so much history in that building. We also visited the Oklahoma City National Memorial, which is one of the saddest places I have ever seen in my life. So much death and despair, but so much hope, too. I highly recommend visiting that landmark when going through that wonderful city.

Normally, the day before a major surgery, the patient has to go to the hospital for some pre-op work. But lucky for me, I already took care of all that. Dr. Moxley's office felt that since I was already in town on the 10th for my initial appointment, and that I was three hours from home, it would be beneficial to me to go ahead and get the pre-op work out of the way. That way, I had nothing to worry about right before my surgery. I was told it would only take about an hour, but it ended up taking over 2 ½ hours, twice as long as originally intended. So many tests! No wonder they elected to have the pre-op work done on the 10th, as opposed to the day before my surgery. They wanted it over with as much as I did!

I was given a set of instructions before my surgery. I was to stop all medications on the Monday before my procedure, including my metformin. Being diabetic, that meant I was gonna have to be really careful about controlling my blood sugar (which wasn't all that hard to do). I also had to stop taking pain meds, especially the week before. (Something about blood clots.) So if I had pain, I just had to grin and bear it. Oy.

I was also told that I had to be at the hospital a little before 5 in the morning. Grr. Those that know me know that I am most definitely not a morning person! (I usually wake up about 9 a.m. or so.) I worked the 11-7 overnight shift for almost 4 years, so one would think I'd be used to being awake at that hour. But I wasn't, which was probably why I switched shifts. Anyhow, I could not fall asleep at all the night before. I slept in fits. I had gone to bed about 7:45, 8:00 p.m. During the night, it seemed like I kept waking up every 45 minutes or so. I suppose part of the reason I kept waking up was because I was afraid of oversleeping, even though I had set the alarm. But a big part of my irregular sleeping pattern was because I still worried about my surgery a little bit. I was still scared, too. Anybody would be, the night before a major life-changing operation. You never know what's gonna happen while you're under the knife. Even though I was in the very capable hands of a wonderful surgeon, I still worried about something going wrong. I guess every person goes through all those mixed emotions. But despite feeling this way, I was ready for the surgery. I wanted my pain gone.

My sister and I stepped outside to get ready for the drive at 4:40 in the morning. (Funny how I was able to remember stuff like this.) I immediately felt tremendously underdressed. I had worn my *Green Eggs and Ham* pajama pants and a pink T-shirt. I had failed to realize until then that I had not brought my hoodie with me on the trip. And oh goodness, it was cold, even though it was only mid-September. Oklahoma weather is a bit fickle, I suppose. It didn't take long for us to get to the hospital from the hotel. Traffic at that hour tends to be a little bit light. On this particular morning, I saw maybe 4 or 5 cards on the highway, which was rather odd, considering it was Interstate 35—one of the busiest highways in the entire United States. But I digress.

Parking at OU Medical Center wasn't so bad, either. During the day, it is horrible. If you've ever been to this medical facility, you'll know it is a humongous beast. There are at least nine floors in this building, and it's an absolute maze—at least 60 rooms per floor. It's all part of OU Health Sciences Center, like I have said, one of the top medical facilities in the country. Four or five buildings clustered together—a children's hospital, some sort of eye clinic, a diabetes research facility, the cancer center, and Presbyterian Tower, to name a few. Presbyterian Tower is where I went that morning. Since I went so early, the parking lot was virtually empty, except for maybe 3 or 4 cars. Something you'll have to understand about Presbyterian Tower—that place is a zoo. If you don't know where you're going, you'll get lost, guaranteed. That had happened to me when I had gone for my pre-op work the last time I was there. I had walked past the same elevator three times—turns out it was the elevator I had needed to use. But on this day, I knew where I was going, so it didn't take that long to get to the check-in desk.

After I got checked in for my surgery, all I could do was wait. It seemed like it took forever to be called to a room to prep for surgery. In reality, though, it was only about 5-10 minutes, which is good for a hospital of that size. The room I went to wasn't exactly a big room. There was room for the bed, a chair or two, and some equipment, but not much else. For a claustrophobe like me, it's not fun. But at least they had a television on the wall to keep me occupied. After getting dressed in that god-awful looking hospital gown that was two sizes too big and funky-looking hospital socks, I waited for the nurse. I couldn't remember her name, but she was so nice to me, as were all the nurses at OU Medical. One of the first things she did was hand me a urine specimen cup. I look at her—and the cup—like she's lost her mind. "But I can't pee in this," I tell her. "I went before I came, and I haven't had anything since last night. I can't pee." She tells me to try my best, anyway. When I ask her why she needed a urine sample, the nurse smiles and tells me, "We need it to do a pregnancy test." I almost fell off the bed. Are these people serious? Me? Pregnant? Psshh. I'm about to have all my female guts taken from me, and you're asking me about babies? Good god. Unless this was the Immaculate Conception, there was no way I was gonna have a baby. It would have been nice, but I wasn't seeing anybody, and you kinda need somebody to do that with, I would think. "Well, it's standard procedure with all of our female patients that are at a reproductive age," the nurse said. Even so, I still thought it was funny—and pointless. So to the bathroom I went. Apparently, I needed to go more than I thought, because I filled the cup halfway. I guess your body can surprise you that way.

After giving my urine sample, more nurses came in for even more blood work. Geez, they didn't get enough blood from me the last time? Why do they need more? But I suppose they needed to make sure everything was spiffy enough for surgery. (It was.) I also got fitted for my IV, too. I tend to be a hard stick sometimes, and it can be hard to draw blood (which was why it had taken 30 minutes the week before when I got my pre-op work done), so it surprised me when the IV went in smoothly. It didn't take long at all. (Maybe it was all the water from the day before.) Then they put on my latex allergy bracelet, my penicillin allergy bracelet, and my two identity bracelets. Whoo, by the time all my bracelets were put on, and my IV was taped up, pretty much the only things visible on my arm were my fingers. I guess they didn't want me skipping out and ensured that I wouldn't. Hah! I wasn't planning on going anywhere, believe me.

Dr. Bishop came to see me soon after that, to make sure I was doing okay. I also spoke with the doctor who was going to be taking care of me while I stayed at the hospital, as well as the anesthesiologist. I also had my blood sugar tested, and it was a little bit elevated, but that was a good thing. Doctors actually prefer an elevated blood sugar right before surgery. It tends to drop during an operation, so a high blood sugar is a good thing. Anyhow, not too long after that, Dr. Moxley came in to see me. Oh, goodness, it's 6 o'clock in the morning, and this woman is way too cheerful. Must be large amounts of coffee or something. Maybe a good night's sleep. Whatever it was, I was glad she was prepared. No sense in having a tired and ineffective surgeon, am I right? We talked for a few minutes, and she did wonders for my nerves. I was a mess that morning—I was cranky, sleepy, and hungry. But something about her demeanor made me feel a whole lot better. I was in good hands, for sure!

I waited a little bit longer after that before I was taken to the surgery holding area. As I was wheeled through the area to get to my spot, I took a look around to see who else was waiting to have an operation. I noticed dismally that I was the youngest patient there. Didn't make me feel too good. I was being surrounded by a bunch of people in their 60's, 70's, and 80's. Bleh. But at least I was relatively healthy (cancer notwithstanding), so I would be able to bounce back from surgery a lot quicker than another hysterectomy patient who might have been older. I at least had that going for me.

At precisely 7:06 a.m., I was wheeled into an operating room prepped just for me. In the room happened to be a couple of nurses, a doctor or two, the anesthesiologist, and of course Dr. Moxley. She asked me if I was ready, and I told her, "As ready as I'll ever be!" She smiled at me and did something I will never, ever forget for the rest of my life. Right before the anesthesiologist administered his medication, Dr. Moxley held my hand and said a small prayer for me. I had never heard of a doctor doing something like that for a patient. Ever. It made me feel so much better. One of the nurses held my hand as the anesthesiologist applied the anesthesia. The last things I remember before I went under was the anesthesiologist putting the mask over my face and telling me to "breathe deeply and smell the plastic".

The next thing I know, I'm waking up 5 ½ long hours later in the recovery room. So much time has passed! But to me, it felt like a few seconds, not hours. The first thing I see after I open my eyes is a blonde-haired angel in the form of a nurse. I have since forgotten what her name was, but she was so, so very nice to me. The first thing she said to me was, "How are you feeling?" Like I had been run over by a garbage truck, I wanted to say to her. "I've had better days," is what I actually said. I couldn't really remember much right then, and I couldn't really think straight. It was probably because I had just woken up from the anesthesia, and I was still groggy. Yech, I hated feeling like that.

I remember looking at the digital clock on the wall, and it read 12:47 p.m. I knew a significant amout of time had passed (5 ½ hours), but it still surprised me when I saw the time. I was told that I hadn't been in recovery all that long, so obviously the surgery itself had taken a while. This could be a good thing. Perhaps Dr. Moxley wanted to take her time to make sure she got everything. Either that, or there was so much to get that she had to take a long time. But I preferred to think of it as Dr. Moxley wanting to take her time. (I wanted to remain positive.) And that was something I truly appreciated.

I ended up spending about 2 hours in recovery. I had a breathing tube inserted into my nose, which I absolutely hated (and it was irritating), so I had the nurse remove it. Whew. Now I could breathe better, and scratch my nose. I also had a catheter temporarily inserted while in surgery so I wouldn't have to get out of bed to go pee. Personally, I think that the person who invented the catheter should be shot. Those things are the most uncomfortable pieces of medical equipment ever invented. You can't move in any direction. At all. But at least it was inserted correctly. I've heard a few horror stores where catheters had been put in wrong. I hear those can be downright painful. But I digress.

I also began to become hungry. I was downright starving. I hadn't eaten since the night before, so it had been a good while. The nurse disappointed me when she told me I couldn't have any solid foods—I was on a liquid diet. What made it worse that I could not have anything at all (ice chips being the only exception) until I was in a regular room. So no, I was not happy at all. My regular room was ready in no time. My body, on the other hand, was not, unfortunately. My blood sugar wouldn't go down, and my blood pressure wouldn't go up. Funny, I figured since I was in such pain and my body had just gone through a major and sudden change, my blood pressure would be through the roof. But it wasn't like that at all. In fact, the same thing had happened to me right after my breast reduction in 2009. I don't know, maybe my body's just weird that way.

My blood sugar and blood pressure were finally brought to manageable levels, so I was taken to a room at 3:30 in the afternoon. Room 756, to be exact. People have no idea how excited I was to be out of recovery. A regular room meant one thing and one thing only to me: food! But I had forgotten that I was on a liquid diet, so I was disappointed when I saw my tray. Instead of seeing a hamburger or something delicious like that, all I saw was a bowl of chicken broth, some jello, some Sprite, and an orange popsicle. Unfortunately, the anesthesia began to wear off then, so I promptly vomited everything I had eaten, except for the popsicle. I was so upset, too. I was looking forward to my meal, and that was what had happened. Dammit to hell.

The pain had truly begun to set in around this time, too. It was as if someone had ripped out my insides. But I guess one could say basically that's what had happened. Part of my insides were indeed removed. Dr. Moxley had explained at one point that the pain was akin to that of natural childbirth, since it was a vaginal hysterectomy. Oh my goodness, now I understood why these women always asked for epidurals! I totally and completely empathize with these ladies for doing the natural childbirth thing. Ouch. I tell you one thing, morphine was my best friend during my hospital stay.

Dr. Moxley came to check up on me while I had been eating. Bless her, she took out the catheter herself. I loved her for that. Now I could finally move around and go to the restroom! It's the small things in life that make us happy, I suppose. But going to the restroom—getting in and out of bed—was so difficult, to say the least. My bed wasn't that far from the restroom—it was a private room, thankfully—but it still took 20 minutes each time I needed to go. And I seemed to go at least once an hour. Bless those RN's, they were so patient with me. Of all the nurses and aides that took care of me, the most wonderful and gracious was the nighttime RN, Derrick. I never met a more patient man. He told me that if I needed anything, regardless of how small it was, I could always call on him. And believe me, I did. I was always calling him for one thing or another: ice water, medication (which I needed several times!), and of course, going to the restroom. At first I was a bit apprehensive about having a male in any capacity help me with bathroom duties, but helped me feel comfortable. He stepped away from the bathroom and let me have my privacy while I was in there. And once I was done, he would help me back to bed. Oh, goodness, getting back into my bed was a friggin nightmare every time I had to do it. I was literally in tears from being in so much pain, and I would need several minutes to regain my composure. This wonderful and compassionate soul waited until he made sure that I was okay before left the room. That was totally awesome on his part. Bless him.

I slept in fits that day, and overnight, as well. I couldn't sleep for more than 30-45 minutes at a time. The intense pain I was going through was preventing me from getting a restful sleep, even with the medication. I was finally able to rest about 3:45, 4:00 in the morning. And wouldn't you know, that was the time that the nurse came in and drew blood. Dammit. The worst part of it was that it took them about 20 minutes because they couldn't find a vein. Pfftt. I told you I was a hard stick. I was so relieved when they got done and left. I was finally able to fall asleep quickly after that and managed to sleep about 3 hours. Progress!

I woke up during shift change and met the new nurse. He told me the doctor said I could eat solid foods now, so that's exactly what I did. I ordered bacon, sausage, eggs, toast, and some apple juice, and believe me, that plate was clean by the time I finished with it! The same thing happened at lunch (cheeseburger and fries) and at dinner (chef salad), too. Hey, don't judge me. After going over 24 hours without any real food, I was starving!

I was discharged from OU Medical about an hour or so after finishing my dinner. Even though I had such wonderful and compassionate people taking such good care of me, I was ready to head home to my own bed. I had ended up staying at OU Medical for a day and a half (but only because my blood pressure didn't want to go up), but I'll never forget the kindness and generosity shown to me. These angels taught me that there are compassionate and amazing people in this crazy world of ours. For every crazy act of violence, there's always a sincere act of kindness. They taught me that even though I was hurting, I was still blessed. I was alive, and I was a fighter. And I was ready to begin this fight and kick cancer's ass.

...klr

Recovery

Recovery from a major surgery such as a hysterectomy often takes a very long time. So they say, anyhow. Dr. Moxley told me that it could take about a year or so before my body would get back to normal. She wasn't kidding.

The pain began when I left the hospital. Speed bumps and pot holes were not my friends that night. The ride home only took 3 hours, but it felt like 3 days. Every time I went over a pothole, it felt like someone was stabbing my abdomen and vagina over and over. The pain was almost unbearable, and I cried so much. It didn't help that I didn't have any pain meds. Oh sure, I had a prescription for some painkillers, but I couldn't get it filled until the next morning. That wasn't going to help me on the way home.

I finally made it home after what seemed like an eternity. Getting into bed was an adventure. It took 20 minutes just to get comfortable. Five minutes after relaxing, the urge to go to the restroom would suddenly hit. It took me 10 minutes trying to find a way to comfortably sit up without pain ripping throughout my entire body. Even then, I was not 100% pain free. Far from it, actually. The fun part was actually sitting down on the toilet. The pain was simply excruciating! No wonder Dr. Moxley said to take my time in getting around, especially when it came to using the restroom. The restroom was my friend those first couple of weeks. Even if I didn't drink anything, I still went. Dr. Moxley had explained to me that this would happen. I had 18 lymph nodes removed, and because of that, the fluid built up and had nowhere to go but out. I'm a lot better now, but in those first couple of weeks, it was as if I lived in the restroom.

Dr. Moxley also prescribed Lovenox injections for a month, in addition to the painkillers. The thought of injections simply terrified me. Those that know me well know that I am absolutely petrified of shots. Just the sight of a needle is enough to send me into a panic attack. I was 25 years old before I didn't need anyone to hold my hand while getting blood drawn. (No, I'm not exaggerating.) So the thought of having to inject myself for 30 days nauseated me. But I got used to it after a while, even if my lower abdomen did look like a pincushion from all the needle marks. I was prescribed Lovenox because I was going to be immobile for a while and was at risk for blood clots. This medication would prevent me from getting them. It didn't mean that I had to like it, though.

One of the bad things about being single and living alone is that you don't have anyone to help you do the small things around the place. Cooking was a nightmare. Breakfast was fun, especially if I wanted cereal. I had so much trouble lifting the milk. And to think, it was only half a gallon. Washing the dishes was also out of the question. I couldn't even load the dishwasher because it meant constant bending and stooping, something I was not allowed to do. And forget about driving my car. I wanted to move it one day from the side of the building to the front, where I could keep a better eye on it. I should've known I was going to struggle when I started to hurt just by putting my seat belt on. I only drove less than half a block, but it felt like 10 miles! So much for taking myself to the store. I couldn't even do that. I was bummed out big time!

The physical healing was slowly taking its time, but the emotional stuff was another story altogether. It seemed like I was always, always crying. One minute I would be happy and smiling, and the next I would just spontaneously burst into tears. My mood swings were just horrible! Happy, sad, cranky, content, irritable…you name it. I was definitely feeling all of those emotions! I had a total hysterectomy after all—EVERYTHING was removed, so that meant no more estrogen and hormones. And I couldn't take hormone therapy because it tends to feed into the cancer. (My tumor was estrogen-fed.) So, yeah…I was kinda screwed. But I tried to make the best of it, and dealt with it in the best way I could.

But the awesome thing through all of this was that I had so many wonderful people supporting me. My wonderful friend Richard came by to see me a couple of days after I came home, and brought me some awesome, freshly-cut flowers from his home garden. It wasn't much, but he took the time out of his day to visit me and lift my spirits. It did wonders for my morale, which was pretty low in those early days. (And to this day, I still have the vase!)

My friend Harlie came to help me, too. The amazing thing about her was that only a couple of weeks before I had my total hysterectomy, she had surgery herself. So she wasn't exactly feeling well, either. Yet, she still took the time to drive me to the store for a few odds and ends, or the pharmacy to get my medications. Not too many people are willing to do stuff like that, especially if they are hurting, too. What an awesome friend.

My aunt Mickey and cousin John were completely helpful and awesome, too. My cousin would often come over to help me throw my trash and re-stock my fridge with bottled water so they would be cold. My aunt, bless her, was 77 years old at the time of my surgery and didn't have the stamina of someone half her age. So it truly touched me when she cleaned my apartment and did my laundry for me. She truly was a wonderful help. My apartment was always spotless after she and my cousin came by! And she occasionally cooked small meals for me. I will love her for life.

Another blessing came in the form of my dear friend Susan. She was so good to me, I can't describe it. She was the only person I knew personally at the time of my diagnosis that had been diagnosed with cancer, so she knew exactly what I was going through, both physically and emotionally. She listened to me when I began crying about my diagnosis. She took me to eat several times, just to get me out of the house and to lift my spirits up. She never, ever let me feel sorry for myself. Not once. Yes, there are other people that were there for me during my time, but there is nothing like having a fellow cancer survivor supporting you along the way.

So many other wonderful amazing people help me during that time, I can't even begin to name them all! I know my sisters were always there, as well as their families. My cousin Enez cheered me up by posting funny things on her Facebook page. And my friends—oh, there are so many of them! I hope they don't feel slighted if I don't mention them by name! But they know who they are, and they ALL hold a special, special place in my heart.

...klr

What Not to Say

There are some things that people have said to me, and they have been wonderful and amazing words of support to me. And then there are those insensitive morons who say all the wrong and idiotic things, even though their hearts were in the right place (but I often wondered where the hell their brains were!). And then there were assholes who were insensitive to me—on purpose. Ugh! But anyway, don't say these things to me, and you will be just fine.

"You can always adopt." Well, no shit. I know I can adopt, dumbass. I just don't need to hear it from you. Most people who have told me this are healthy women with children of their own. They've never had to deal with the pain of having uterine cancer, and having to go through the bigger pain of needing a total hysterectomy before your first child is born. I feel robbed already, and I don't need to hear those words. It may not seem that way, but to me, it feels condescending. You don't know unless you've been through the same thing. So don't tell me to adopt. Please.

"You can have sex all day long, and you don't have to wear condoms or worry about getting pregnant." Umm…what? OK, that makes total sense. I don't use condoms anyway, because I'm allergic to latex. (That's sure to scare the guys away!) And about that whole sex thing…yeah, ok. Like I need to think about sex, considering my hormones are totally out of whack and my sex drive goes through the roof all the time. Of course, not having anyone to do that with doesn't help, either. (And no, having toys to use is no substitute.) If I had someone, it would be completely different. But honestly, cut me some slack!

"I wish I could have your problem. I'm tired of dealing with all these periods!" Uhh…excuse me, stupid, but that is one of the most insensitive and most ridiculous things you could ever say to me. It's as if you don't think my ordeal really is all that major. Of

course it is! Cancer is never minor. People die from it all the time. I was a lucky one. I survived it. But you have no idea how much I would love to experience the cramps, the bloating, all that other stuff if it meant not having cancer. So please don't ever tell me you wish you could have "my problem". Be careful what you wish for, as they say.

"You don't look sick at all." That's because I have taken good care of myself post-surgery and followed my oncologist's advice. And my cancer was caught early, so I didn't need any chemotherapy or radiation. Cancer itself doesn't make you look sick—it's the treatment you have to endure that makes you look that way. I didn't know I had to look a particular way to show I was fighting cancer. I didn't get that memo.

"You need to stay at home and relax." Perhaps this may be true. But a little fresh air never hurt anybody. Besides, I needed to move around a bit. I had a serious case of cabin fever that was driving me crazy! And doctors do recommend a little bit of exercise. Of course, I'm not gonna be a total moron and overexert myself, thereby hindering my recovery. I'm not that stupid. But exercise—in small parts—does wonders for your health, not to mention your emotional well-being.

A lot of people don't know what to say when someone they know personally is diagnosed with cancer. Stuff like what I just described isn't exactly wise to say. When in doubt, don't say anything. That is all.

...klr

Stage 1a, Grade 2

Thursday, October 4, 2012 was a particularly cloudy day. Rain was part of the forecast and was expected all afternoon. This worried me, because I hate traveling in bad weather, regardless of whether I'm driving or not. In this particular case, I was not.

Dr. Moxley told me that she wanted to see me in her office two weeks after being discharged from the hospital. For me, that meant the 4th day of October. My friend Dinah graciously offered to drive me to Oklahoma City for my appointment, which was good, considering I did not yet have clearance to do much of anything. So in the middle of the morning, we take off to the state capital of Oklahoma.

The drive there just about killed me. Not physically, of course, but emotionally and spiritually. For 14 days, I was in the dark about my cancer. So many thoughts ran through my mind. Did Dr. Moxley get it all? Was she thorough enough? What stage was it? Did it spread? Would I need more treatments and lose my hair? Dinah did her absolute best to keep me engaged in conversation, but my mind still wandered. I wanted this day over with already!

It wasn't all that cold when we left Vernon, but when we stepped out of the car at the cancer center parking garage, that blast of cold air hit me hard! I was tremendously under-dressed in just a shirt and a pair of shorts. Yeah…not a bright idea, Kathy. No wonder I was being laughed at. I learned my lesson about being unprepared!

I checked in at the front desk and waited. I had never been so damn nervous. Yes, I was a bit apprehensive (to say the least!) during the drive to OKC, but it was nothing compared to what I was feeling then. And it got worse when I got called to an examination room. It almost was to the point of nausea. Thank goodness Dinah had gone into the room with me. I don't think I could have gone through this alone. I probably would have gone nuts without her.

Dr. Moxley came in after a few minutes, and asked how I felt. "Quite nervous," I said. "And anxious." She smiled and assured me I wouldn't need to be for too much longer. She took a look at my incisions from the surgery—one in my belly button, two on my sides above where my ovaries once were, and one near the vaginal opening (where my cervix was once was), all of which hurt like hell—and examined my vagina. She said I was healing quickly, which pleased her immensely. She also explained the incisions would eventually heal and fade away, and my body would go back to normal. I asked her how long that would take, and she told me, "Most women bounce back after about a year." Wow. A whole year. Twelve months of experiencing aches and pains I had to endure, and that was if I didn't have any more complications.

Before letting me go, Dr. Moxley said she wanted to see me again in six weeks to see how I'm healing, and asked if I had any more questions for her. Well, of course I had a question. A very important one! "What stage am I at?" I asked, staring up at her. Dammit, I just had to know! "You are at Stage 1, grade 2. Very early." Meaning what…? "It means we caught it in time before it could do any more damage." Is this a good thing? "You don't need any chemo or radiation. We got it all during the surgery. You're not going to lose that beautiful hair of yours." Really?! "Really," she said with a big smile. "I'll see you in six weeks," she told me before leaving the room.

No more cancer. Wow. That was something. I was in remission. My goodness! I never heard better news in my whole entire life. Ever.

I had only smiled when Dr. Moxley revealed what my stage and grade were, so I didn't think I was going to have much more of a reaction than that. Wrong. I sat up to get dressed, looked up, looked down, inhaled, exhaled, and…cried. I had never cried so much in my entire life (except for when my mother had died). I covered my face with my hands in an effort to keep from crying. But it didn't help—the tears flowed harder. I simply could not stop crying. I had never been so relieved in my life, I just cannot explain it. The hard part was over. I did it. I beat cancer. In fact, I kicked it in the ass! I couldn't believe it. So there I was, sitting in an office exam room, half undressed and with a paper cover hiding my unmentionables, crying my eyes out, and one of my dearest friends giving me a gigantic hug of support. No words were said then—no words needed to be said. It was exactly what I needed to push forward and get dressed—and begin the process of starting the next chapter of my life.

I asked for and received a copy of my pathology report detailing all the results from the insane amounts of tests they ran on my female bits. There it was, in black and white: *endometrial adenocarcinoma, FIGO Grade II, Pathologic Staging T1a.* The tumor was confined to the endometrium and had only superficially invaded the myometrium. Basically what this means is the tumor was limited to the inner lining of the uterus and had barely begun to stretch to the middle lining. Whew. I was grateful that it wasn't anything more than that. This type of cancer is a slow-moving one. I was told that a majority of the times, the cancer is found early enough where surgery is the only thing that is necessary. So I was one of the lucky ones. To this day, I have my pathology report framed and on the wall. It serves as a reminder of what I faced—and beat.

In speaking to me, Dr. Moxley said that based on the staging, my age, and overall health, I had a 3% of recurrence. If I don't get it again after 2 years, then that chance goes down even further, to about 1 ½ %. Amazing. Simply amazing. I think I can live with those odds. I don't mind it at all. And if I go five years without a recurrence (which is what I am shooting for), I'll be considered cured of cancer. Yay! I think I can live with that.

The only thing I would have to do now is make frequent trips to Oklahoma City for the next 5 years: once every three months for two years, and once every 6 months for three years after that. After 5 years, I believe I'll only have to go once a year for the rest of my life, but to my regular gynecologist. Small inconvenience perhaps, but I don't really care. If it means staying cancer-free, I'll drive anywhere.

I alternated between crying and napping on the drive home. It was an emotionally and physically exhausting day for me. I still had trouble wrapping my mind around the fact that I was now a cancer survivor. Not a victim, mind you, but a survivor. Sweet, sweet words to hear, indeed.

...klr

Hair Loss

It was a relaxing day at home—really, that's pretty much the only thing I could do without hurting so damn much. It was perhaps less than a week after visiting Dr. Moxley and receiving the awesome news. I had been showering for several days and noticed that I began losing strands of hair over that time. I didn't really think anything of it, because people tend to lose small strands of hair all the time. No big deal, right? That was what I had thought.

I had taken a shower early that Friday morning. While rinsing out my hair, I pulled out a small chunk of hair. Normally, I would not be freaked out, but with everything that had been going on, I panicked. It was a good chunk of hair. The back of my hair had been itching like crazy for some time, and for the life of me, I could not figure out why. I guess my scalp was irritated and was shedding the hair follicles.

It wasn't until later that afternoon that I definitely knew something was wrong. I was watching TV and the back of my head began to itch again, so I scratched it. When I did, I felt a smooth spot, where I had earlier pulled out the chunk of hair, that I should not have been feeling. I immediately headed for the bathroom to check for any other spots. I couldn't really tell, so I took a picture of the part of my head where I had felt the smooth spot. Holy crap, it was bald. Why the hell was it bald? It wasn't supposed to be this way.

I took a second (and more thorough this time) look at my pathology report, to see if I could figure out why I was losing so much of my wonderful hair. As I finished reading the section about my ovaries, I saw the words "consistent with polycystic ovary disease". Huh? What did that mean? So I did what any other normal person would do: I looked it up.

It turns out that polycystic ovary disease makes a woman's hormones to go out of whack and causing all sorts of problems, most of which I had. Some of the symptoms include acne, fertility problems (though I never really tried to find out, seeing that I was single and unattached), irregular periods, voice changes, body hair where you don't want it, and of course male-pattern hair loss on the scalp. (And though it doesn't always happen, it can occasionally lead to endometrial cancer.) Oh. So maybe that's what had happened to me and my hair. So I called Dr. Moxley.

First thing Monday morning, I called her office. The nurse explained to me that occasionally women experienced hair loss after their hysterectomy. But she didn't think it was due to the polycystic ovaries. She explained to me that it may have been directly related to the surgery. *How*? I asked her. She told me that it might have been as a result of being laid flat on a hard surface, such as an operating table, for a long time and not being able to move. That seemed to make more sense to me. After all, the hair loss was only in one spot (albeit a large one), and it didn't happen until after the surgery had taken place. But it still freaked me out, and I was afraid the nurse was wrong, and even said so. She told me that if the hair loss continued, I was to call them back and they would do some tests during my next visit. That was some relief to me, I suppose.

Even though I knew what may have caused it, the hair and bald spot still bothered me a little. Okay, it bothered me a lot. I tried not to think about it, but it was still there. Every time I combed my hair, I could feel the bald spot. So I did something totally and completely drastic: I made an appointment with a hairstylist and had my hair cut off—all of it. I went all G.I. Jane on my hair! I couldn't believe I had done something this wild. And it was something I couldn't take back—it was a done deal, and I would have to wait until my hair grew back. Oh, well.

As it turned out, I ended up not losing any more hair. Yes, I occasionally lost the runaway strands, but it was nothing like before. So, yeah…no wonder people questioned my move. But it was okay after all, because not having much hair has done wonders for my hot flashes. And I have saved a fortune in shampoo and other hair products. Hah! The haircut ended up making my huge amounts of gray hair stand out, but I'm okay with that, too. It goes to show I'm a fighter.

...klr

Going Back to Work

The trouble with living alone is that sometimes you're bored and get a little bit lonely. I would sometimes go to the store, just for the specific purpose of being around people, not necessarily because I needed something (which I usually didn't). Of course, I couldn't necessarily spend a lot of time there because my energy would be totally sapped. But I at least got some fresh air, and that helped me out a lot.

But it was definitely no substitute for being at work, where I would be around people all the time. Okay, so some of these people drove me nuts sometimes, but they were generally good people, and I genuinely liked working with them. I missed my co-workers a great deal, and I wanted to see them again. So what could I do, especially since it hadn't yet been 8 weeks since my surgery? Then it suddenly came to me.

I called Dr. Moxley's office one morning and spoke with one of the nurses, Allison. I positively begged her to let me return to work on the 29th of October, two and a half weeks ahead of schedule. She looked at my file and said she didn't think it would be wise to return to work just yet. Then she asked me what I did for a living, and I explained my job title and where I worked, and she said, "Absolutely not. We can't risk your health that way, and set your recovery back."

I wasn't ready to give up, though. I was determined to return to work, no matter what. "Well," I said, "can I at least do light duty? I wouldn't be working directly with patients. I'd be put in the back office and would work on the computer." Allison thought for a minute. "That sounds like something we could agree to," she tells me. Whew. I was gonna get to go back to work early, after all. Yay me. Now all I have to do is get the paperwork in order, which took a few days, but I got it done.

The thing about working for the state of Texas is that there is a process you have to go through in order to get a significant amount of time off. If you request more than 3 days off from work due to a medical condition, you have to fill out paperwork under the Family and Medical Leave Act (or FMLA, for short). The wonderful thing about FMLA is that it protects your job if you get sick. You can't get fired if you don't come in to work, as long as that paperwork is on file. But it can also be a huge pain in the butt, too, just to get the paperwork filled out by the doctor, especially if you're three hours away from their office. And getting the Fitness for Duty certification filled out can be a hassle, too. Without it, you can't return to work. But thankfully, I was able to get my Fitness for Duty form returned to me rather quickly, and my date of return rapidly came up.

October 29th was a Monday, and I was just way too excited to sleep, so I woke up early. I couldn't help it. I was finally gonna get to drive to work! Yay! So many happy thoughts and emotions went through my mind.

To me, that morning went by so slowly. I was just so anxious for 1:30 to arrive so that I could get ready for work. But it seemed that every time I looked at the clock, only 5-10 minutes would pass. It was like that all morning long. But eventually the clock hit 1:30, and I got ready for work. I can even remember what I wore that day: navy blue shirt, a long-sleeved white shirt under it, blue jean pants, Nike sneakers, and of course, my Dallas Cowboys beanie (my hair was still pretty much non-existent). At 2:07 p.m. (yes, I looked), I headed out towards the state hospital.

As I pulled into the parking lot, I suddenly became nervous. I don't know why, but right then I wanted to turn right back around and go home. Seriously. I don't know what came over me, but I didn't think I could face my co-workers. So much time had passed since we had last seen each other, I didn't know what we would say. I didn't know how they would react to my radical change in appearance and attitude. I didn't want them to feel sorry for me, but I didn't want them to be totally ignorant of what had happened to me, either. I just didn't know. But I had to go forward and began my way to work.

I had almost forgotten how far the walk was from the parking lot to my unit. Whoo, that walk wiped me out and thoroughly kicked my ass! It seemed like it took forever to get to the back office, but I finally made it. The first thing I did was turn in all my necessary paperwork. Then I visited with a few of the office people, who were pleasantly surprised but happy nonetheless to see me. Then I went to see my bosses, who were happy to see me, too.

After that, I had to wait until a little after 3 o'clock to see any of my co-workers. Most of them weren't expecting to see me until the middle of November, so to say they were pleased was an understatement. A lot of them were afraid to hug me, though. They thought that if they touched any part of my body, it would hurt me. I had to reassure them several times that small hugs would not hurt me, as long as they didn't try to squeeze me too hard. So after getting past the initial fear of hurting me, they would give me hugs and ask how I was feeling and how the surgery went. They also asked how I managed to deal with the emotional trauma of the cancer. Day by day, I would tell them. That's all I can do. Several people also asked if I had to do chemo and/or radiation. (I knew that cutting off my hair was gonna have unexpected reactions!) No, I tell them. It was caught early enough that surgery was the only thing necessary. But at least they asked questions and didn't assume anything.

For the most part, my first day at work was a good one. I spent most of the shift in front of the computer, doing office work. There were a couple of insensitive boobs who didn't (or refused to) understand why I decided to come back early and felt I should have stayed at home. But I didn't care about them. They didn't matter to me. What mattered to me was the love and affection shown to me by those who truly cared.

...klr

Faking It

There are so many things that people should lie about and fake all the time: their age, weight, perhaps money, sex (women are really good at faking orgasms—sorry, guys, you had to know it's not genuine ALL the time, right?), crying, to name a few. But there are some things you should never lie about. Cancer is one of them.

Another thing you should never do is accuse someone of faking their cancer to get attention, unless you have proof. You shouldn't say something like that just because you can't stand the person. Back up your words.

Why do I even bring this up? Well, because it has happened to me, sadly. It saddens me because I never expected it to happen. And it was deeply, deeply hurtful.

It was a Sunday when I found out what was being said about me. Yes, this person has an extreme dislike for me (for the life of me, I just don't understand why, but oh well), but that was absolutely no excuse for saying I faked having cancer just so that I could get attention. Bitch, please. Like I would want attention. Most people who know me rather well know that I don't like attention. In fact, attention embarrasses the hell out of me. I go out of my way to avoid it. People know that I'm naturally shy and can't bear to have so much focused on me. No way.

Another thing: it's rather difficult to fake cancer like the type I have, dumbass. You can't fake any type of cancer, when you think about it. Believe me, it's very difficult. (It still boggles my mind that people are able to pull it off, though.) You can't fake the ultrasounds that revealed the location of the cancer. You can't fake the biopsy that was done. And you most definitely can't fake all the blood that gushes out of the vagina that ultimately leads to the cancer diagnosis. But some people don't understand that. They believe what they want to believe, and nothing will ever change their minds. And that's just too bad.

I could never, ever fake the painful journey I have been through. Anyone who's had a total hysterectomy like I did knows that this is one of the most painful surgeries to endure. It's something I would never wish on anyone. After struggling to get in and out of bed every day and even falling out of it a couple of times (that was no fun at all!), being sick from the sudden body change, after struggling with severe bouts of depression, not to mention never being able to have children—who would put themselves through something like that? Not me, that's for damn sure! No way. And I'll never understand why anyone else would, either. There's a special place in hell reserved for those who pretend to have cancer for attention or monetary gain. It's absolutely ridiculous.

Like I said, I'll never begin to understand why this was said about me. Why I was accused of faking my cancer battle—I can't put into words how hurt I was. It almost caused me to walk out of work the night I found out. But a wonderful friend convinced me to say. He told me that as long as I knew the truth, and my doctors knew the truth, that was all that mattered. The hell with what everyone else thought or felt. And that's true. What matters is how I feel. Nothing else.

I won't say who this person is or how I found out. They don't deserve that much attention. I will, however, pray for their soul, because obviously they have no love in their heart. But I will say this, though: karma always comes back to haunt you. Always.

...klr

Peaches

It's been said that dogs are very smart and very perceptive animals. I firmly believe this to be true. Allow me to explain why I have come to change my mind about these precious creatures.

When I was a little girl (and my family can tell you this), I couldn't stand dogs of any type. I was absolutely, deathly afraid of them. I would refuse to be in the same room as a dog, and would refuse to go outside whenever I was at my sister's house because I knew her dog was there in the yard. I could never figure out where this unnatural fear of canines came from. I have never been attacked by a dog before in my life. Cats, yes, but I never feared them. Go figure.

As I got older, my unnatural fear of dogs subsided, and I have grown to respect them. I still don't really feel all that comfortable around them, but at least I can be near them and not totally freak out. Now I think they're wonderful.

Anyhow, I saw a story on *Unsolved Mysteries* once where they profiled a group dogs who could detect cancer in humans just by going up to them and sniffing them. Their trainers would place several lumps of human tissue (or something like that) close together, and would inject one of the lumps with cancerous cells. The dogs would sniff the air, and every single time they did the test, the dogs would calmly walk toward the lump with the cancer cells, and would not move from that spot. The trainers would even move the cancer lumps to different spots. Never fooled the dogs. Not once. I thought this was simply amazing, but I didn't think this could actually happen in real life. But that was before Peaches came along.

Peaches was a wonderful, wonderful Chihuahua owned by my friends Richard and Tipton. She was a precious, precious dog, but could be a little diva sometimes, and most definitely temperamental! Every time I would go over to Richard and Tip's house, I would see Peaches roaming around, barking at something or somebody. Peaches is no longer with us, poor thing, but before she died, she had gone deaf and would not hear you call out to her. She always seemed to like to bark at me, but she never tried to do anything to me. Then one day, her attitude toward me seemed to change.

My friend Boston and I have birthdays that are close together, so we decided to have a joint birthday party at Richard and Tip's house. Of course, you know Peaches had to be roaming around, protecting her "turf", so to speak. I didn't see her right away. But after walking around for a few minutes, I felt a tiny ball of fur at my feet. I looked down and I saw two big brown eyes staring back up at me. "There you are, Peaches," I said to her.

I figured Peaches would start barking at me again and be on her way. But this canine diva surprised me. Everywhere I walked, whether it was inside or outside, Peaches was hot on my trail. She kept sniffing me and licking my legs. And if I sat down, she kept trying to jump in my lap. "What is up with this dog?" I would ask. "I don't know," someone would say. "Maybe she's in heat or something." And she was possessive, too. Anytime someone got near me, she would growl. Not a high growl, but a low-pitched one, one you could barely hear. Wow, Peaches. She was like my personal guard dog that night. She never, ever left my side and never tried to stop sniffing me. What an amazing dog.

I never really thought about that night, until I was at a party a few months later. People started talking about their dogs and about how the dogs were very perceptive. It suddenly dawned on me—this party and Peaches' antics occurred on the 19th of August—a full five days before I had received my cancer diagnosis. Holy crap. Peaches was able to detect the cancer and knew I had it before I did. Wow, that's all I could say. Told you Peaches was an amazing dog.

...klr

Side Effects

Before and even after my surgery, Dr. Moxley had explained to me that I would have plenty of side effects. Some she told me about, some I had to find out on my own.

She told me that without a uterus or ovaries, I would never be able to have children. Well, that was definitely a given. Everyone knows you can't carry a baby without having a uterus. She also said since my ovaries were taken out, I would go into immediate and sudden menopause. Because the menopause had happened so suddenly and at a young age for me (32 years old), I would have such bad reactions. I thought she was completely exaggerating. Hah! Nope! The hot flashes were so horrible, I can't explain it. I was so, so sick from the nausea, I could hardly eat anything. I even lost a few pounds. (For a diabetic like me, that can be dangerous.) I also had to take 2 showers a day sometimes because my body had poured out so much sweat. What stunk was that I could not be put on hormone therapy from the loss of estrogen because Dr. Moxley said most hormone therapy medication tends to feed into the cancer. Dammit. I had no luck.

I had fallen off my bed not too long after I had surgery, and I landed on my right hip. Because of that, I now have problems with my right hip whenever there is an extreme weather change, such as high to low temps, or vice versa. And the only way that the pain subsides is when I take medication, which I don't like to do and only helps about 75% of the time, anyway.

Another major casualty of my surgery happens to be food. Not only is it a casualty, it's a major, major disappointment. I have had a lot of trouble—a lot!—with food since my surgery. For one thing, I simply cannot tolerate lettuce at all, in any way, shape, or form. (Of course, it doesn't stop me from eating it. I just pay for it later.) The first time I experienced problems was the day after my

60

operation when I had that chef salad. From the first bite I took to the last one, I had severe stomach pains. It felt like someone was stabbing me in the gut. I figured that it was a one-time thing, but each time I ate lettuce (a Big Mac, tacos, sandwiches), I experienced the same exact problems. Dr. Moxley explained to me that I would always experience problems with not only lettuce, but with all leafy greens. So there goes the occasional salad. That's a shame, because I love salads.

Bread has made me incredibly nauseous, too. I can't eat more than one slice before getting the urge to vomit. So sandwiches are out. Pizza is, too. But funny enough, I have no problems with breadsticks. Go figure. And sometimes even smells nauseate me, even if they didn't bother me before. Fried chicken—the smell of it, anyway—is unbearable to me, as are beans, and hell, even mustard. But I guess it depends on how I'm feeling that particular day. Sliced cheese gives me fits, too, but shredded cheese is okay. How odd. I guess it's in the way cheese is made. And don't get me started on bacon. I simply cannot stand the smell of bacon cooking. Therefore, I can't eat bacon.

About the only two things that do not give me problems are baked chicken and pasta. So, in the time since my operation, I have lost weight because there are not too many foods I can tolerate lately. And when I do eat, I don't eat as much because I get full more quickly. Sometimes it's hit or miss when it comes to food. I have to take each day as it comes. Dr. Moxley says that I won't always be like this. My remaining organs just need time to adjust to overcompensate for the loss of my reproductive system. I certainly hope so. But it's a small price to pay, though, to be cancer-free.

...klr

November 15, 2012

As I previously said, I have to go see Dr. Moxley once every three months for two years, once every six months for three years after that, and yearly for the rest of my life. My first such visit of this type occurred in the middle of November.

I had learned my lesson from the previous visit to OKC and came properly dressed. Considering it was colder than it was in September, I'm glad I remembered the hoodie and the blue jeans.

I filled out my paperwork at the front desk and waited to be called back to a room. The wonderful thing about the Stephenson Cancer Center is that you never, ever have to wait long for a room. In my case, I only had to wait about 10 minutes. I got my vital signs checked and my weight measured. Vitals were good, and I had even lost a couple of pounds. Yay! No post-hysterectomy weight gain for me! Whew! Dr. Moxley did a Pap smear and said everything looked good down there. She answered all of my questions, especially about taking medicine to help with the severe hot flashes. At first she was reluctant to give me anything because it would tend to increase the chance of a recurrence. I most definitely did not want that, but I also did not want to suffer through the awful bouts of hot flashes, either. So after discussing a couple of things, she decided to put me on Aygestin. It's a type of hormone therapy, but she says that it won't feed into the cancer. Oh hey, in that case, sign me up. Anything that can help, I will gladly appreciate, believe me.

After my appointment with Dr. Moxley had ended, I got measured by two nurses. Umm, what? Every time I would see Dr. Moxley, my legs, arms, and abdominal area would be measured to check for lymphedema. Lymphedema happens sometimes when a person has had surgery to remove cancer and lymph nodes are removed. Since the lymph nodes have been taken out, fluids don't really have anywhere to go. Sometimes it'll go out the same way that urine and bowel movements do. And sometimes, the fluid will stay inside your body and will build up, causing your arms and/or legs to swell up, causing numbness or pain, or difficulty in moving around. Well, according to the nurses measuring me, I most definitely did not have lymphedema because I was shrinking from the last time I had been measured, during my initial visit. What a tremendous relief. I had enough issues dealing with the cancer, it was nice to know that I didn't have to deal with that, too. Whew.

    I was given a release to go back to work at full strength. Dr. Moxley felt I was ready enough to resume full and normal activities. I still had to be careful as far as my abdominal area was concerned, but it was nice to know that I could finally begin to move on with a new chapter in my life.

...klr

<u>Why I Relay (blog entry)</u>

(If you have read my blog, you'll recognize this entry. I thought I should include it here. Relay for Life is so important to me, especially now! ...klr)

I've always been a big supporter of anything related to cancer survival and research. I only had an uncle who died from cancer, but I was only eight years old, so I don't really remember him all that much. My friend Susan was diagnosed with breast cancer last year (2011), and after going through grueling treatments, she's in remission. Good news, indeed. But I never thought that my experience with cancer would go beyond that. (It's one of those things where you feel detached, until it happens to you.) But life had other plans.

I was diagnosed with uterine (or more commonly called endometrial) cancer in August 2012. I was stunned, to say the least. I had been having excessive vaginal bleeding, which led to a pelvic exam, Pap smear, and biopsy. It was during these routine examinations that the cancer was found. I simply cannot stress enough the importance of these yearly exams. Too often, women go years without these simple (but lifesaving) tests. The discomfort is not fun to experience, but it beats the hell out of the alternative.

I had a total hysterectomy in September 2012, and my wonderful oncologist explained that my cancer was found at Stage 1a, Grade 2, one of the earliest stages. I did not have to do any chemotherapy or radiation, praise the good Lord, but I did lose some hair. So I went ahead and chopped off the rest of it. A bit drastic, I know. But it serves as a reminder of what I've gone through. Dr. Moxley says I will have to be monitored closely for the next five years, but I only have a 3% chance of recurrence. I think I can cope with those odds.

It is my sincere hope that one day this type of cancer, as well as all types of cancer, will be eradicated. If we pull together and support the American Cancer Society and other organizations like it, cancer will one day be history.

Kathy Rodriguez

Survivor, endometrial adenocarcinoma

Babies

Babies and small children are such blessings. They are so innocent and pure, a reminder of all that's right with the world. The things they do to make you smile and laugh—it's just so wonderful!

I am ashamed to admit that when I was younger, I didn't like kids all that much, unless it was family. Small children in stores and restaurants annoyed the absolute bejesus out of me. And I most certainly didn't want any of my own children. Absolutely not. I didn't even want to date a guy who had kids. Then I began to realize that this behavior was rather selfish. There were so many wonderful guys I have met that have small children of their own. Who knows how many potential relationships I have missed out on just because I didn't want to love someone else's child. There was an absolutely amazing guy I met a couple of years ago who had a son who was about 3 years old, and the child was simply adorable. How could I not love someone like that? Unfortunately, my opinion of children changed too late to have any type of relationship with this guy. And that forced me to change my way of thinking.

Some precious babies came into my life that have mellowed me out, too. My nieces' and nephews' children have meant so much to me! Natalia, Adrian, Isabel, Sophia, Sebastian, as well as my other nieces and nephews are all beautiful little angels! Every time I see one of them, it just brightens up my whole day. And I love to make them laugh and smile, especially little Sophia. She's a little diva and difficult to please! She was a year old when I was recovering from my surgery, and did not like people who wore hats or beanies, so before I would head over to see her, I always took off my beanie. I love her that much, I was willing to do that for her. I love all of my "babies" so much, I can't describe it. They are my life.

These precious, amazing babies made me realize that I really did want to be a mother. I had so much love to give to a child. So, so much. I couldn't wait to have children of my own. My mother had instilled so many values and morals in me, and raised me right. I had wanted to pass that on to a child, and make the world a better place. A bit idealistic, I know, but hey, I had wanted my child to have my mother's spirit and determination.

As the years went by, however, and I got older, I began to lose faith that I would ever give birth to a child. I still had a glimmer of hope that I would, though—I even had a couple of names picked out in case I had any: if I had a girl, her name would have been Faith Elizabeth or Ashleigh Brooke, and for a boy, I had picked out Adam Joseph or Anthony Paul. I tried believing in myself and hoping that I would eventually become pregnant. After all, my mother was 39 years old when she had me, and my grandmother was 41 when she had my mom. But somehow, deep down, I just knew that I was never going to truly experience the joys of motherhood, as much as I had wanted to do so. And it turns out, I was right.

I have heard some women who have had hysterectomies end up freezing their eggs and eventually having someone else carry their baby. I figured I could do that, even though I knew it would be expensive. But it was something I was willing to consider. After all, I might meet someone one day, and we might want kids. However, Dr. Moxley said that my ovaries were too badly damaged, and had to be removed. My eggs couldn't be saved. That was simply devastating! It was one of the most heartbreaking things I had ever heard in my entire life. I know, there was a small nugget of knowledge in the back of my mind that there would never be any children in my life that would be biologically mine, that would call me "mom". But to hear your doctor tell you that there is absolutely no chance whatsoever you'll ever give birth to anyone—well, it hurts. It hurts a lot. It leaves a deep void like no other, trust me.

What makes me sad about all of this is that I see so many women that don't deserve to be mothers give birth to 4, 5, or even 6 kids. I've even seen them mistreat the ones they already have, and announce to the world that they're pregnant with another one. Oh, that drives me positively insane. I've been out in public, and I've seen women slap their kids for crying about wanting a toy. They tell their kids no, there's no money, but yet they'll turn around and buy beer and cigarettes. Yeah…that makes sense, lady. A lot of sense.

There's also a young woman that I know of (several of them, to be honest with you) that has publicly claimed to love her kids and talks about them all the time, but privately wants as little to do with them as possible, preferring instead to go out to clubs and partying, or spending time with her significant other. I know of another woman who dropped off her son with her ex-boyfriend and since then, she has not seen her boy, who is now in his 20s. Kinda sad, when you think about it. Meanwhile, there are so many women in this world who would love to have children and can't. They either have trouble conceiving (like my dear friend Ashley) or have had cancer, which has robbed them of the chance to bless the world with a child.

It doesn't really seem fair somehow. People who deserve to be mothers, can't seem to catch a break. And then there are some women who have no business reproducing and pop them out like a Pez dispenser. There seems to be no logic whatsoever. It's like we're being punished for something that we didn't do or something that is out of our control. We have enough problems, and we don't need to have this added stress.

There are those that tell us to adopt children, since we can't have any. While I think it's a lovely and noble idea, it's still no substitute for childbirth. And only people who have been in my position can truly understand how I really feel. Because no matter what you do, no matter how many nieces and nephews you have, there will always be that void caused by cancer that nothing can ever fill.

…klr

Emergency Visit

The thing about uterine cancer and hysterectomies is that occasionally you'll have unexpected complications. I had been recovering as expected, but I still wanted it to speed up a little. I wasn't complaining, though. That was before I started hurting again in December 2012.

I had been feeling okay, but out of nowhere, I began having such severe stomach and abdominal pains. No matter what I did (or didn't do), I was hurting. The pain was so, so sharp, I would literally be in tears, and doubled over. I would eat something, I would be in pain. I drank something, I was in pain. I sat down, stood up, walked, lay down…you name the activity, I was feeling the pain. It was a very sharp, shooting pain, like something or someone was stabbing me in that sensitive area. The pain I was feeling was the exact same pain I was feeling right before and right after my surgery, except that I didn't have all the vaginal bleeding. It worried me, because I thought this meant that my cancer had returned. Oh, no, this just could not be happening to me. My life was just starting to go back to normal, and I was beginning to adjust to life again. How could cancer be coming back so soon after receiving such an excellent diagnosis? So I called Dr. Moxley's office in a panic, and I was asked to come in as soon as possible.

I pretty much had one thought on my mind during my drive up to Oklahoma City. I kept thinking that my cancer had come back—or rather, it had never really gone away in the first place. It felt like I was part of the 3% chance that would be unlucky enough to get a recurrence. I did not like this idea at all! No matter how hard I had tried, I could not get the idea out of my head that cancer had returned. It seemed like the harder I tried to think positively and push the thought out of my mind, the worse the feeling got. I just could not get to Oklahoma City fast enough.

Dr. Moxley asked me how long I had been experiencing my severe pain, and I told her that it had been going on for about a week and a half at that point. She did a physical exam, and it seemed like every time she touched something, it would hurt like hell. It would not feel good at all. But despite my pain, Dr. Moxley told me that I had absolutely nothing to worry about.

Honestly? I had nothing to worry about? Then why the hell was I always in pain? "Well, it's not cancer coming back," Dr. Moxley tells me. Well, that's a relief, I tell myself. But it still didn't solve the problem of what was really going with me and my body.

Dr. Moxley explained to me what my problem was, and it turns out, it's really not all that uncommon among women my age who have had hysterectomies. My issue that brought me to the emergency visit was that I was having muscle spasms in the vaginal area brought on by tension. Huh? Vaginal tension? I've never heard of something like that. My wonderful oncologist tells me that it can often be brought on by stress, both physical and emotional, and it can often be relieved by massages and exercises, as well as medication. So she gives me a prescription for two painkillers, and advises me to relax and do some exercises. Okay, I tell myself. I can most definitely handle that. And if it continues, she says, I could always come back for another visit. So I head back home to Vernon with peace of mind that I knew—finally—what was going on with my body, and that it wasn't cancer!

I was halfway home from Oklahoma City when it suddenly dawned on me what Dr. Moxley was trying to tell me when it came to "exercise". Oh, hell! No wonder the woman had a small smile on her face when she talked about getting that exercise. Oh…Kathy's vagina isn't being used enough, so that's why it has tension. Hmm, I thought to myself as I drove home. How is this gonna work? I'm not dating anybody, and I don't have any "friends with benefits" (my mother certainly didn't raise me that way). A co-worker of mine told me the next day that I should buy myself a "battery-operated boyfriend". That would solve my issues. Why couldn't I have thought of that idea before? Duh!

Luckily for me, my dear friend Kara is a consultant for a

company that sells adult products. What a lifesaver she was! I certainly didn't want to go online to buy this stuff, and going to an adult store didn't really feel right, either. At least when you shop at home, you can shop at your own leisure. That appealed to me. So now that I talked with her, I'm set up. The products I saw are not on the cheap side, but you get what you pay for!

Since then, I have not had any issues with tension or anything like that. I see this as a good thing. I took Dr. Moxley's advice and learned to relax, not to let things bother me. Really, that's all I can do.

...klr

Love and Loss

It's been said that if you are lucky enough, you'll find someone who will mean the world to you, someone who will take your breath away and give you a reason for living. You will find someone to spend the rest of your life with, someone to love. Me, I haven't been so lucky just yet in my 30-plus years of living. It's probably because of my past hang-ups and fears, as I have said previously. Because of that pain and rejection, I told myself that I would never let anyone push through the walls I had built up, that I would never, ever love anyone again. But that was before *he* came into my life.

I have to admit, I wasn't really looking for anyone to spend time with, much less someone to fall for so hard. Then I met him. It was a few years ago.

The first time I saw him, I remember thinking to myself, *wow, what a really good-looking pair of eyes!* They were the most striking set of blue I had ever seen in my life. Honestly, it was the only thing I noticed about him that day. It wasn't until the next couple of times I ran into him, that I noticed the rest of him, and it wasn't too shabby, either. Because he was such a good-looking fellow, I simply could not bring myself to talk to him. I wouldn't know what to say to him and how to say it. I was just that shy around him. But the funny thing is, he started talking to me first. I don't know why; maybe it was because I didn't try to hit on him like all the other females he came across. Because he started becoming friendly, that put me at ease and allowed me to open up. And we became fast friends. I got to know him better—I found out things about him, such as his name (that was of utmost importance!), his age, his birthday, among other things. He's always been so nice to me, and has opened up to me, when he normally wouldn't otherwise.

I don't know exactly what made me truly fall for him.

Maybe it was because the interior was more wonderful than the exterior. I just love that kind of personality. I truly feel that we are so much alike. We've gone through some of the same things, and have some of the same beliefs and values. Of course, it doesn't hurt that he's kinda easy on the eyes, too. Hah!

So what's my problem? I don't know, exactly. Like I have said, I'm extremely shy. But once I get to know someone, I'm more open with them. He's different, though. I can't quite put my finger on it. He's simply so amazing to me. We've gone through similar things in our lives—heartbreak, stuff like that—so we could be kindred spirits, so to speak. We'd be absolutely perfect together, I just know it.

But unfortunately, I am letting my past dictate my present (and potential) happiness. My self-esteem is so bad, I find myself wondering what the hell he would want with someone as plain as me. I'm not the prettiest, thinnest, or tallest. I can't offer him the opportunity to have his own children someday. I know that this is important to him, and the fact that I can't do that for him really hurts inside.

At the same time, I don't know what's going through his mind when it comes to me. Does he think good things? Or are they bad? I don't know. But because I won't say anything to the man, I'll always be left wondering.

At the same time, he could say something, too. Sometimes I feel that if he was truly, truly interested in me, he definitely would have said something by now. If a guy was honestly interested in a girl, he would let her know and pursue her. If not, he ends up saying nothing. Nothing at all.

But then again, he might be pretty shy, too. He might have a painful past, just like I do (but not the same kind of pain), and that prevents him from ever opening up his heart to another woman. And that's sad, because I'm a terrific person. I know I'd make him happy. Thing is, though, he has to make that decision on his own. I can't force him to decide to love me. If I do that, I risk losing his friendship. And that's not something I wanted to experience.

Unfortunately, I never told him how I felt, and now he's with someone else. Someone who is better for him than I ever could be, and I'm ok with it all. After all, when you truly care for someone, you want nothing but happiness for them, even if it's with someone else.

...klr

Valentine's Day 2013

When most people think about Valentine's Day, they think of chocolates and flowers andfancy gifts. Not me. I had one thing on my mind—endometrial (uterine) cancer.

It's February 14th, 2013, and for me, that meant another 3-month checkup with Dr. Moxley in Oklahoma City. Let me tell you—I was quite nervous. I always am before these visits. I don't know why, but I always seem to think the worst. I always feel like I'm going to get bad news or something like that. And it's a feeling that never goes away, no matter how much time passes.

After the last trip I made to Oklahoma City, I decided that I would at least stay overnight this time. Six hours in a car in one day is just too much for me. I wasn't gonna put my body through that again. No way.

I got up early that day so that I could get ready and take care of some last-minute things. I was actually organized this time! Yay for me. I left at about 11:30 that morning to Oklahoma City. Why did I leave so late, especially since this city is three hours away? Well, my appointment wasn't until mid-afternoon, just like all of my appointments are (except for the first one, which was way early in the morning). It's no coincidence that my visits are so late in the day. I have my appointments set up at this time of day because I have no desire to get up so early in the morning just to get to an appointment that's three hours away. No sir.

It seemed that the closer I got to Oklahoma City, the more nervous I became. I did not want to go to this appointment at all. But I knew I had to get it over with. So, despite my misgivings, I got out of my car, and walked into the building and up to the second floor.

I didn't even have the chance to finish filling out my

paperwork before I got called to an exam room. Geez, I didn't even get the chance to write down any questions I might have wanted to ask the doctor. I sure hoped I would be able to remember it all.

I should have known something was up when they called me less than five minutes after arriving at the front desk. After I got put in an exam room, I waited. And waited. I was by myself for about 30 minutes or so. I even managed to finish my paperwork—and promptly fell asleep. The first people I saw were the two nurses who measured me for signs of lymphedema. The measuring usually happened after the appointment, not before. But oh, well. I was still shrinking from the weight loss, so I still didn't have the lymphedema. That was a plus. One less thing to worry about.

Dr. Moxley came in right as the nurses finished up their measurements. Poor woman, she was just getting over an issue with a sore throat. Welcome to the club, I felt like telling her. I was also recovering from a severe throat infection that had almost developed into strep throat. No bueno.

According to Dr. Moxley, I was healing nicely from the surgery. Perhaps a little too well, it seems, she tells me. I still remained cancer-free (which was all I really cared about), but I had developed some scar tissue in the vaginal canal. She said that it was not cancer, but she still wanted to cut it out and send it off for testing. The process took about 5-10 minutes, but with the discomfort of having tools inside my hoo-ha and cutting something out (and fully awake!), it felt like 5-10 hours.

That was pretty much the extent of my check-up. I had been having a couple of problems with vaginal discharge, and Dr. Moxley said it was because of the extra scar tissue. She said that since the tissue was taken out, I should not be developing any more problems. It turns out that she was right—the vaginal discharge went away, and the tissue did not have any cancer cells in it. That was good news to hear, indeed.

I went back to my hotel room and ended up going to dinner at Denny's. After I finished my meal, I went back to my room and spent the rest of the evening relaxing and watching television. I was watching a re-run of *Reba* and I burst into tears when I heard the last line of the theme song: "I'm a survivor". I couldn't help it. But they were tears of joy. And it's true. I am indeed a survivor. I know that there are some people who think I'm making too much of a big deal about my battle with cancer. Well, it kind of is a big deal. Your life is never the same. For the rest of your life, you carry the label "cancer survivor". But that's okay with me. I would not have it any other way.

...klr

Mom

    I'm not gonna lie—when my beautiful mother died back in 2009, it was simply devastating. My mother was my life. I cannot put into words how much that wonderful woman meant to me, how much I loved her. So yes, her death hit me really, really hard.

    So many emotions went through me as I continued to grieve and mourn her loss. Sadness, pain, anguish, grief, heartache, agony—those were just some of the feelings I experienced because of her death. I felt like I had lost my best, best friend. I suppose she was indeed my best friend, once you think about it. There was nothing she didn't know about me. She knew all of my thoughts and feelings and emotions. If I was feeling something, she definitely knew about it. She had absolutely no problem expressing to me how she felt about something I was going through, and always gave me a little advice, whether I wanted it or not. That was just her way; she was never, ever afraid to voice her opinion to anyone.

    I guess the first time I truly felt the enormity of her loss was in August 2012, the day I received my cancer diagnosis. After getting off the phone with the doctor's office, I had burst into tears. The first person—the very FIRST person—I had the urge to call was my mom. I ached for her—I can't explain how badly I wanted to be with her right then. I wanted her to hug me, to let me know that everything was going to be okay. There is nothing in this world that is like a mother's love and touch. It was something that I could have used right then. It pained me to know that I could not have that from her.

    I guess this was also truly the first time that I was angry with my mom for leaving me. I don't think I had felt like that before about her. How dare she leave me when she knew that I was gonna need her? Didn't she know what was going to happen to me? Didn't she know how to stop this cancer from coming? Seriously, how could she be so selfish? This was the one time that I really needed her to be there for me, to be by my side. And she wasn't there for me when I needed her. I was quite upset about that one, believe me.

Then I got to thinking one day. My mother has never, ever, ever left my side. Not once. And she has most definitely been there every step of the way since my cancer journey began way back in August 2012. I felt her presence when I visited Dr. Moxley for the very first time. And she was there for me on September 19, 2012—right there in the operating room at OU Medical Center. And, as wild as it may sound to some people, when I was told that I was at Stage 1a, Grade 2, I could feel my mother hugging me in support, and celebrating the wonderful news with me, right there in the exam room.

Something I forgot to mention: the day of my surgery, my mom was there with me. I was being wheeled into the holding area to wait for an operating room to open up. In the corner of the area, there was a Hispanic woman in a bed. She looked exactly like my mom—same haircut, glasses, facial features. She saw me, smiled, and waved. I smiled and waved back at her. I simply could not get over how much she looked like my mother. The resemblance was striking to me. Anyway, as I was being wheeled to the operating room, I passed the corner. I looked over to wave at the lady again, but when I looked, all I saw was medical equipment. I asked the nurse what happened to the lady, and she told me there was never anyone there. As adamant as I was in my belief that my mom was there, the nurse was just as adamant in hers that my mom wasn't there. But I maintain to this day I saw her.

So in a sense, my beautiful, sweet mother has *never* left me. She's always been by my side, just like a mother would do anytime her baby needs her. So how could I get mad (or stay mad, for that matter) at this wonderful, fantastic woman? She may not be here in the physical sense, but she's most certainly there for me in spirit. And it gives me great comfort knowing that no matter how many trips to Oklahoma City I make, she's right there, watching over me. I can't ask for a better guardian angel.

...klr

Famous People and Uterine Cancer

When I was first diagnosed with uterine cancer, I started thinking about other people who might have had this terrible disease. I don't know anyone personally that has had this particular type of cancer. I figured that I would have, but I didn't.

In doing some research on this subject, though, I did find that there have been celebrities that have had this type of cancer. There have even been some that have actually died from it, which saddens me.

The first person I actually thought of that has had uterine cancer was The Nanny herself, Fran Drescher. I remember hearing way back in 2000—around that time, anyhow—that she had been diagnosed with uterine cancer. I remember much was written about this when it happened. I also remember that she had written a book about her experience with cancer. The thought of the book always interested me and I had been wanting to read it for quite a while, simply because *The Nanny* was always one of my favorite shows. When I got diagnosed with the same disease, I promised myself that no matter what, I was going to buy the book and read it. So about a week after my surgery, my copy of her book came in. As I was reading her book, my heart just broke. I simply could not believe what I was reading. It was just hard to imagine that she had to endure 2 years of symptoms and had been misdiagnosed by 8 different doctors. How hard that must have been to go through for her. But the good thing was that uterine cancer is a very slow-moving cancer, so she didn't require anything other than surgery. The cool thing was that she had a sense of humor about everything, which is important. Without humor, you don't really have much.

Another person I had read about during my research was Queen Mary I of England. Today we have so many advances in medical technology, so uterine cancer can be completely cured if it's caught early enough. But during Queen Mary's time in the 16th century, not much could be done to help a woman if she got sick from cancer. In fact, cancer of any type was pretty much a death sentence. In Mary's case, legend has it that she may have died of uterine cancer, or it might have instead been ovarian cancer. But one thing was for certain: she had been very, very sick and in lots of pain for a good while. Some people might have called it karma because of all the religious persecutions that occurred under her command. (They called her Bloody Mary for a good reason, I suppose!) But still, nobody deserves to go through torture like that, regardless of what they've done in their lives.

When I was growing up, I remember watching Shari Lewis and Lamb Chop. I thought it was pretty cool how she used a lamb as a puppet. I had never really seen something like that before, so it caught my attention. And they were funny, too! I loved it. But I remember hearing back in 1998 that she had died. I don't think I had ever learned what she had died from—I just knew that she was no longer with us. So imagine my surprise when I learned she had been diagnosed with uterine cancer and died two months later. But she didn't actually die from the cancer. She was getting treated for that when she developed pneumonia. The pneumonia was what had killed her. Who knows? If she hadn't gotten the pneumonia, she might have even survived the cancer. But that's how life goes sometimes.

If you've never really paid attention to the movie *Gone with the Wind*, then you have probably never heard of Evelyn Keyes. She had several movie roles during her prime (even acting in the same movie once with the great Marilyn Monroe). But I don't believe that any of her roles were as big as that of Scarlett O'Hara's sister Suellen in *Gone with the Wind*. I remember that character very well. Scarlett steals her sister's boyfriend from her and marries him. Anyhow, I had no idea that Evelyn had died way back in 2008, and I certainly didn't know she had been diagnosed with uterine cancer, something that had eventually killed her. (Of course, complications from Alzheimer's disease didn't help her, either.) It certainly saddened me, to say the least.

My mother liked to watch *Designing Women* back in the day,

and she got me to watch the show and like it, too. Her favorite character on that show was Julia Sugarbaker. Oh my, how my mom just loved her! She like how Julia always spoke her mind and was never afraid of anything or anybody. (I guess you could say my mom was exactly like Julia!) I was sad when I had heard Dixie Carter had died in 2010. I knew she had died from endometrial cancer, but at the time, I had no that endometrial cancer was the same as uterine cancer. (Just goes to show how uneducated I was!) I also noticed she hadn't been diagnosed with it for very long before dying.

In doing my research of celebrities who have had uterine cancer, I noticied that the older females tended to be the ones that unfortunately succumbed to this terrible disease. Perhaps it might have something to do with their age. Or maybe it's because they have a diminished immune system that keeps their bodies from being able to fight off the cancer. I honestly don't know. I do know one thing, though: cancer does not discriminate against anybody. It doesn't care about how many Oscars or Emmys or Tonys or Grammys you may have won. If it wants to attack you, it will attack you, no matter what.

...klr

Uterine Cancer: Signs and Symptoms

According to an article published by the Mayo Clinic, endometrial (or uterine) cancer is defined by the fact that it begins in the uterus, and cells form on the endometrial wall. There are several signs and symptoms that women experience which often lead to a cancer diagnosis. Sadly, women often ignore these things until it is almost too late.

One of the major signs of uterine cancer is vaginal bleeding after a woman's gone through menopause. It's most definitely not a normal or pleasant thing to experience. That's why women are taking themselves to the doctor when they go through something like this.

Some more symptoms that can indicate uterine cancer include prolonged or bleeding between periods. That's what happened to me. I had a period that ended up lasting almost exactly two miserable months. Yeah, that's bad. Most normal periods tend to last only a few days. Mine lasted a few weeks. If something like this happens to you…get yourself to a gynecologist IMMEDIATELY!! And don't put it off for another day. It could make a huge difference as to how much treatment you will end up getting.

It's also bad if you experience any type of pain down there, such as pain during sex, or pain in your pelvic area. But it doesn't always indicate cancer. It's still worth checking out if you're always, always experiencing that type of pain. Better to be on the safe side, I suppose.

There is no way of predicting whether or not a woman will get uterine cancer. Lack of family history doesn't necessarily mean anything. Look at me. I had only two family members get cancer before I did, and they weren't even direct relatives (an uncle and a male cousin). There are several circumstances that factor in to whether or not cancer will occur. Of course, just because these factors are present, it doesn't mean you'll get cancer. But at least you'll know what to look for. The most important thing—the *most* important thing—to remember is that you know your own body better than anyone else does, and if you even suspect that something might be a little bit off, then it would be beneficial to you to get yourself checked out. Intuition is the best tool in this fight. In fact, your life might depend on it.

...klr

Uterine Cancer: Staging and Basics

There are a few things to remember when it comes to uterine cancer. A majority of the time this cancer is caught early, because one of the symptoms is unusual vaginal bleeding. Women hate regular vaginal bleeding, and don't want to go through it any more than they have to. They want it to go away as soon as possible, and would be willing to do anything to get it to stop.

Since uterine cancer is found at an early stage, most of the time a hysterectomy is the only thing that a woman will need. But it's important to remember that there are three types of hysterectomy that are performed: subtotal (where only the uterus is removed, but not the cervix); total, like I had (where both the uterus and cervix are taken out); and radical (where doctors go in and take out the uterus, cervix, and part of the vagina—ouch…this type of hysterectomy must be quite painful!). Occasionally, but not always, you'll have your ovaries and tubes removed (that particular procedure is called a salpingo-oopherectomy, what a mouthful to say!). Why a doctor would remove a uterus but not the tubes and ovaries is beyond me. But I learned that once you have your ovaries removed, you go into surgically-induced menopause. It's been said that surgically-induced menopause is worse than regular, natural menopause, so doctors try to avoid it if possible. So I can understand why a doctor would leave one or both ovaries inside. (Surgical menopause was not fun, believe me!)

There is more than one method of how a hysterectomy is done: open abdominal and laparoscopic-assisted. An open abdominal hysterectomy tends to take longer to recover from than a laparoscopic-assisted one. The hospital stay is about 3 days or so for an abdominal surgery, as opposed to an overnight hospitalization from a laparoscopic operation. And the pain from a laparoscopic surgery won't be as bad as the abdominal one, because they don't cut you wide open. So the recovery time is quicker. However, most of the time, the hysterectomy is done abdominally, probably because it would be easier for the doctor to see if the cancer is present elsewhere. I guess it just depends on each woman's situation and what the doctor is comfortable with doing.

Of course, as with any type of surgery, there are risks that you have to consider when undergoing a hysterectomy. Some are harmless, and some can be serious. Most of the time, though, the benefits far outweigh the risks. I'd rather deal with small aches and pains than having to deal with the torture of cancer.

As with other cancers, uterine cancer has four different stages: I through IVB. Each stage tells you how far your cancer has spread. My cancer was at IA, so it hadn't spread beyond the endometrial wall. You don't want your cancer to be at Stage IVB. The prognosis isn't very good at that point. But that doesn't mean miracles can't happen. Cancer isn't a death sentence now, like it was back in the day.

Until I had been diagnosed with cancer myself, I didn't know that in addition to staging, cancer cells were grouped according to grades. There's GX, G1, G2, G3, and G4; GX is the lowest grade and G4 is the highest. The lower the grade number, the less aggressive the cells are. If you're at a lower grade, your chances are better for recovery. Lucky for me, I was at grade 2, so I was in really good shape.

Depending on what stage your cancer is at, your chances of survival may be excellent. If it is at Stage I (like mine was), your chances are at least 88%, according to the American Cancer Society and the National Cancer Data Base. There are also several types of uterine cancer (which I most certainly did not know about), according to the ACS, the most common type being endometrioid adenocarcinoma, which is what I had. Adenocarcinoma is by far the most curable, compared to the others. But just because you have another type that isn't adenocarcinoma, it doesn't mean you can't beat it. Remember, you are a fighter!

...klr

What to Do and Where to Go

The most frightening thing in the world, or perhaps the most frightening moment, can be when you hear your doctor tell you "you've got cancer". I know that for me, when I heard those words coming from Dr. Winfrey's office, it was easily the most painful set of words I ever heard a medical professional say to me. It honestly felt like my world had ended. I truly felt like I was going to die. I had people that loved me, but I felt alone, that no one could understand what I was going through. I didn't know what to do, where to go, or who to talk with about anything. Everything was just so overwhelming to me! But luckily I was able to get myself together, and everything started to turn out fine.

Don't be afraid to ask questions. Doctors don't mind if you asked about your diagnosis. In fact, in some cases, they encourage you to take a proactive approach. Whenever I visit Dr. Moxley, the front desk always gives me a small notecard where I write down any thoughts or concerns I might have. It's really helpful to me, because sometimes when I'm talking to her, I'll forget what I'm thinking about and won't ask. With the notecard, Dr. Moxley can address anything and everything I have written down.

And definitely don't be afraid or nervous about asking for a second opinion. If your doctor is truly skilled at what they do, they'll understand why you feel the way you do, and respect your decision. Hell, in some circumstances, certain insurance companies might even require the second opinion. Don't stop until you are satisfied with the answers you are given.

It's also important to remember that you don't have to cope with this disease alone. You have your family and friends that will love you and support you. Believe me, you'd be surprised how much people will be there for you. I know I was surprised to see how people came together to do things for me. It's a pretty neat thing to see, I tell you.

Even though that support is nice to have, it's nothing compared to be surrounded by fellow survivors that know what you are going through and can give you some advice like no one else can. So find yourself a support group to get through your journey. If you are on Facebook (as I am), go find the group "My fight Against Uterine Cancer" and request to be added as a member. There are so many wonderful fantastic women that have been my supporters and my cheerleaders. No, they are not doctors or anything like that, but they have been through the same, tough journey that I have, and know exactly how I feel on my good days and my bad days. They are very non-judgmental, and have answered every single question I've asked since I joined the group. Honestly, they are true lifesavers. I really don't know where I would be without them.

The American Cancer Society and the National Cancer Institute have a wealth of information on your type of cancer. They can lead you to the right information and can answer any question you might have. In addition to information, the American Cancer Society can also provide you with assistance during your treatment. They can provide you with a hotel room to stay in when you go for your visits. They can also give you rides to appointments if you need them. They provide so many services, it's simply impossible to name them all! ACS has been so wonderful to me during my journey, I can't even begin to describe it. That's why I try to give back and participate in Relay for Life events. It's my way of paying it forward.

Even though what Lance Armstrong did during his cycling career was wrong and he deserved what he got, it does not take away from what he has done for cancer treatment and research. From what I've read, LiveStrong has raised over half a billion dollars for cancer. I've had the extreme pleasure of working with this wonderful organization. I simply cannot put in to words how amazing they have been to me during this time.

There are so many things you can do in order to cope with your cancer diagnosis. Try to get as much information as you can so that you can be well-informed when speaking with your doctor as far as treatments go. But don't get so overloaded with information that you begin to feel overwhelmed and don't know what to do. Then you'd be right back where you started. And that wouldn't be good.

One of the most important things to remember is that above all, you are a survivor from the moment you hear those three little but devastating words: "you have cancer". And it's okay to cry when you are having a bad or tough day. Don't feel guilty for having that bad day. You have traveled a tough journey. Even the strongest of people can break down every once in a while. It just means that you have been so strong for so long. And remember: you are a fighter. No matter what, no one can ever take your spirit and determination to fight away from you.

...klr

Epilogue I: Pushing Forward, One Day at a Time

As I write this last chapter, it's just now been six months since I got that call that would forever change my life. I'm not going to lie to you: the road I have been traveling since August 24, 2012, has not been easy. Quite the opposite, actually. It's most definitely been, without a doubt, the most difficult journey I have ever made. I most definitely would not wish this heartache and pain on anybody, not even people I don't like all that much. But you know what? If I had to go through all of this again, I would probably choose to do it, anyway. Why? Because if I hadn't gone through this difficult phase, I wouldn't know what I know now. And I would not trade that for anything.

For one thing, I didn't know that there were so many wonderful and amazing people in my life that truly care about me and my well-being. They have truly made my life so much more enhanced, not that it wasn't enhanced enough already. And I have learned that deep down inside, people are truly, truly compassionate human beings. It warms your heart.

I also learned that uterine cancer is tremendously under-researched and under-recognized. Breast cancer and cervical cancer tend to get more press and more recognition. And that's totally commendable and understandable. They deserve all that recognition, and so many women (too many) have lost their lives to these terrible diseases. But uterine cancer has been called the "forgotten" cancer. People haven't really paid attention to it all that much. And you know what? They really, really need to take notice. Most folks don't know (and I'll have to admit, I was one of them) that uterine cancer is the #1 gynecological cancer. You're more likely to get it than other "women's" cancers, in others. And not enough people know about the symptoms. Women don't pay enough attention sometimes to their bodies to know that something is wrong. Even if they know that something is amiss, they ignore the warnings because they don't want to go through the discomfort of all the testing that comes with all of this. That gung-ho attitude needs to stop, and needs to stop *right now*! Thousands of women die every year because they ignored everything until it was too late. That is heartbreaking.

Something else that I learned through all of this is that September is Uterine Cancer Awareness Month, and that peach is the designated color for uterine cancer awareness. I have bought several peach-themed things, including an awareness bracelet (kinda like the pink bracelets you see for breast cancer) you will always see me wear. Wearing the bracelet has paid off a little bit. People have asked me what the color means, and I am happy to tell them all about uterine cancer. I suppose that it is my way of educating others about this deadly disease. Perhaps that is my new purpose in life—to educate others and making this cancer more noticeable, the way it deserves to be.

Above all, I have learned that I am most definitely not alone in this fight. So many people are in my corner and are wanting to fight this battle with me. I've also learned that no matter what happens, I'm a fighter. Will my cancer come back? I don't know. Chances are, it probably won't. But whatever happens, I'm ready.

Kathy Lee Rodriguez

February 27, 2013

10:42 p.m.

Epilogue II: Getting Better Yet! (an update)

So much has happened in the 3 ½ years since I wrote the last chapter. Where on earth do I begin? For one thing, I've graduated to 6-month checkups. Haven't come close to a recurrence (knock on wood), and next year, God willing, will mark 5 years being cancer-free. How awesome that would be...talk about being blessed! Two years after getting cancer, my precious grand-nephew Joshua was born. He means the world to me! For years after my cancer diagnosis, I couldn't bring myself to hold a baby or deal with anything baby-related. That was before Joshua Ray Maldonado came along on June 8, 2014. From the first time I held him in my arms, I just fell in love with him! He has helped me so much in the healing process, I can't even explain it. We have an unexplained bond that can never be broken. Yes, I love all of my nieces and nephews equally, but there is just something about Joshua. A friend of mine said once Joshua was probably sent specifically to help me heal from the emotional wounds cancer inflicted on me. I totally believe that to be true...no doubt in my mind at all!

I switched to another department where I work, so I no longer work with the people who helped me through my initial cancer fight. My new coworkers know almost nothing about what I went through, unless I just happen to tell them. Some of them tell me they admire my strength. I don't know about having any strength, but I am glad they know my story. But I will never, ever forget those that helped me in the beginning.

Joshua has a new baby brother now. As I am typing this, Misael Guillermo is just about 8 months old. I love him so much too! He has an amazing smile and laugh. It just makes me fall in love with him over and over again. He's something else, that's for sure! Cancer may have taken away my opportunity to become a mother, but I will never be without the love of a small child. And there are other ways to become a mother, thanks to Joshua and Misael and their sisters and cousins. Through them, I learned that I do not have to give birth to love a child. Besides, the guy I end up with might have children of his own. And those children might not have a mother to love them, right? Right now, I am 36 years old, so chances of meeting someone who does not have children is pretty slim. And I am okay with that.

    About a year before my cancer diagnosis, I began having serious trouble with my shoulder, to the point that I could not use my arm. I was undergoing treatment for that problem when I was diagnosed with cancer. After that, my shoulder problems kinda took a backseat. Shoulders seem rather minor compared to cancer ravaging your organs. I had problems with my neck, too, but I didn't think anything about that. As it turns out, I should have. Around the time of my third anniversary of being cancer-free, I began to have troubles with the same shoulder again. I could not use my arm at all, it was so numb. I was sent to an orthopedic surgeon, but bless his heart, he didn't really think that it was to the point of needing surgery. I was adamant that I was hurting. He didn't think the same way I did, but to his credit, he asked me, "Has anyone ever looked at your neck?" Well, no, they hadn't. I didn't see any correlation between my neck and my shoulder problems. Sure, I had had neck spasms for years, but I thought it was because I had very large breasts. When not even the breast reduction cured them, I knew there was something wrong with my neck. But I honestly thought that the neck and the shoulder were two separate issues. Not necessarily, the orthopedist said. He ran some tests on my neck, and sure enough, I had a badly herniated disc that was going to require surgery at some point. So I figured neck surgery would happen soon enough. Wrong. The orthopedic surgeon said I needed to see a neurosurgeon. Fair enough, I thought to myself. Because of the way my medical insurance is set up, I had to see a neurologist first, so that I could get a referral. The first neurologist I was going to be sent to didn't really have a good reputation, so I asked to be sent to a second one. The second neurologist didn't deal with neck issues, so I couldn't go to her. Meanwhile, I'm thinking to myself, what kind of doctor doesn't work on the neck? But oh well. So I was sent to a third neurologist. Major mistake on that. I knew I had heard this doctor's name before, but I couldn't remember where I had heard it. When I saw this guy's face, I immediately knew where I had seen him before. And that was not a good thing. Years before I went to see him so I could figure out why I kept having headaches. I saw him for six months, and he did absolutely nothing for me, except to push medications. So I quit seeing him, and still had the headaches. Anyway, I digress. During this particular visit, he did next to nothing except ask me questions. Even after looking at the report the orthopedic surgeon wrote, he still said there weren't any issues and couldn't understand why I was in tears. He was rather condescending to me, and ordered physical therapy and more medication, both of which failed miserably twice before. He told me to come back in 2 months to see how his orders were working, and he would renew the therapy after that. I knew in my heart and mind that physical therapy was not going to work, so I tore up the orders for PT and medication and refused to go back to him. So I asked my doctor to send me to a fourth neurologist, one that would actually do something to help me. While waiting for an appointment, I had surgery to remove a benign cyst from my wrist, something that developed as a result of the neck issue (at least that's what the orthopedist said). I recovered from the wrist procedure before I got an appointment with the neurologist. He was amazing! He told me I definitely had a problem, and I needed to be operated on as soon as possible. The herniated disc wasn't going to get better, he said, and it was gonna cause even more problems. So I was sent to a neurosurgeon, and I had neck surgery almost a year after I began to have problems again. Honestly, getting cancer was easier. Only three weeks had elapsed between diagnosis and surgery. This other issue took a year! But one thing cancer taught me was to be patient when things didn't go my way. It also taught me to be proactive in my health, and not to be satisfied with one answer if I felt it was not the right one. Now I'm on the mend, and I am finally starting to feel better. I still have issues, of course, but nothing like before this surgery (whose medical term is anterior cervical discectomy and fusion—say that 3 times fast). And no more blinding headaches!

My precious nephew Jeremy was diagnosed with leukemia six months after I was diagnosed. He tells me doctors never really told him what stage he was, but he spent several months undergoing grueling chemotherapy and radiation. If you look at him now, you would never know he was sick. He never had a hospital stay in his entire life, never got a major illness...yet he had cancer, anyway. Doctors told him the reason he was able to bounce back so well from the leukemia was because he was so healthy in the first place. I thank God all the time that Jeremy is in remission. He has my mom's fighting spirit in him, after all.

My brother-in-law Jose died two years ago. Bless his heart, he didn't take care of himself until it was too late to be able to reverse what his body was doing to him. He was one of my biggest supporters, and was always there for me. And I'll never forget him for that.

I am still unmarried...not even dating anybody. It is to the point that people wonder if I'm gay—which I am not, by the way. (Not that there is anything wrong with that!) I am too shy when it comes to expressing to a guy how I feel, and it's cost me a couple of times. But that's okay. I know the right guy is out there for me. It's just taking a little extra time for me to find him, that's all. As they say, good things come to those who wait, right? After all, my cousin didn't get married until he was almost 42 years old. So there is hope for me yet!

My brother Ismael finally got released from prison almost 3 years ago. He went in when I was 8; he got out when I was 33. He served 25 years altogether. Yes, he made some serious mistakes, but he feels as if he has learned from them, and has done everything in his power not to make them again. The only thing that made me sad he served his entire sentence was that our beautiful mother did not live to see him released. One thing that kept her going for so long was that she wanted to see him get out. But he told me one time that he wrote to her, telling her not to hold on just for him, that he would see her someday, even if it wasn't in this lifetime. She died not too long after that. My sister Rachel and I went to pick him up when he was released, and it felt like something was missing: our mom. But Ismael said he wasn't sad at all; mom was there in spirit, and was celebrating with us. In the years before my brother's release, my mom and I talked about where we would take him to eat when he got out. She said she wanted to take him to McDonald's and order him a Big Mac meal, large-sized with a Coke. I never told anyone, especially my brother, this dream of hers. When we got into my car, I asked my brother where he wanted to eat, since it was close to lunch time, anyway. Without hesitation, he tells me Mickey D's. Wouldn't you know, he ordered a large-sized Big Mac meal with a Coke. He later told me he felt compelled to go there and order that exact meal, even though Rachel and I would have taken him anywhere he wanted and would have paid for it. We would have even gotten him a steak and/or lobster. But no, he wanted the burger. So that's what we got him. See, I told you our mom was with us that day. In a way, he was sharing a meal with her. He was the only son she had, so there was a special bond with him that she didn't have with us 4 girls. Of course he is gonna be sharing something with her, even if she wasn't there in the physical sense.

My body is not the same anymore, as you can obviously see. It takes a lot more energy to do the things that used to require little effort. I can thank uterine cancer and my herniated disc for that. When I was visiting with the neurosurgeon about scheduling surgery, he told me that for a disc to be that badly damaged, I had to have had some sort of traumatic event occur in my lifetime. So I think back to July 31, 2004, the day of my car accident. That's the only thing I can think of that my body went through, I tell the surgeon. He then tells me the accident is the most likely culprit. But it's weird, I told him, because I didn't have any symptoms right away. Even the extensive testing I went through after the crash didn't reveal any problems. The only thing that popped up was the insane amount of back spasms I had, which I don't even have anymore since I had my breast reduction. But I can't be mad at the drunk driver who nearly killed me and my family. I forgive him for what he did, but that doesn't mean I will forget. At the same time, though, I can't help but think how my life would have turned out if I had never been in that accident. I might be a mother, even though I don't know that I would have wanted that life. And I would not be having neck-related issues, might be able to use my arms correctly. But it's all good, though. I would not have learned the lessons I did because of my cancer diagnosis, and I might not have learned who's really a true friend to me. I learned patience. I learned kindness. I learned empathy. I learned not to take life so seriously all the time. So many lessons I have learned in the past 12 ½ years that I would not have learned otherwise.

Kathy Rodriguez

12:03 a.m., November 4, 2016

Credits

I went to so many sources to get the information I have given. Gotta give credit where credit is due! So here goes! (check out the websites, too!)

"Uterine Cancer—Staging and Grading." *Cancer.net.* American Society of Clinical Oncology. *N.D.* web. 10 Feb 2013.
Mayo Clinic Staff. "Endometrial Cancer." *Mayo Foundation for Medical Education and Research.* 4 Dec 2010. Web. 10 Feb 2013.
"Hysterectomy: 6 Things Women Should Know." *WebMD.* 25 Jun 2012. Web. 13 Feb 2013.
Wikipedia, the free encyclopedia. Wikimedia Foundation, Inc. 8 Feb. 2013. Web. 10 Feb 2013.
"Survival by stage of endometrial cancer." *American Cancer Society.* 17 Jan. 2013. Web. 22 Feb 2013.
Drescher, Fran. "Cancer Schmancer." Warner Books, Inc. 2002.

LiveStrong Foundation
www.livestrong.org

American Cancer Society
www.cancer.org

Choose Hope
www.choosehope.com

Stephenson Cancer Center at the University of Oklahoma
www.oumedicine.com/cancer

Kathy's Cancer Journey
http://kathyscancerfight.blogspot.com/

MD Anderson Cancer Center
www.mdanderson.org

National Cancer Institute
www.cancer.gov

www.ingramcontent.com/pod-product-compliance
Lightning Source LLC
Chambersburg PA
CBHW070327190526
45169CB00005B/1785